THE AMA   !L

BACK
PAIN
CURE

JUSTIN PRICE

The BioMechanics (Books)
San Diego, CA

Praise for The Amazing Tennis Ball Back Pain Cure

The BioMechanics Method Tennis Ball Techniques (TBTs) described in this book have helped millions of people around the world find relief from chronic back pain. Here's a sample of what people are saying about this amazing back pain cure:

"I searched many years to find a natural remedy for my degenerative arthritis and back pain. I was headed for the operating table when I found The BioMechanics Method TBTs. Within the first few weeks, my back pain was totally under control and I was functioning normally again."
- *Sally Gonzalez, Rancho Penasquitos, California*

"As a personal trainer specializing in helping people with chronic pain, I work with bad backs on a daily basis. The tennis ball techniques are especially useful to 'calm down' overactive and tight muscles. From neck to feet, they are a very simple and effective solution for chronic muscle aches and pains."
- *Hector Garcia, Personal Trainer, Barcelona, Spain*

"I used the simple tennis ball techniques in this book to alleviate the hip, back, and knee pain I had as a result of years of competitive sports. They are easy to use and have helped me more than I could have imagined possible."
- *Lisa Bogiwalu, Netball Player/Coach, New Zealand*

"There is nothing like feeling lower back pain day after day. After a few short weeks of being diligent with the tennis ball techniques my back pain is gone! These techniques are easy, fast and efficient. Thanks, Justin, for all your help."
- *Kim Fiddes, Edmonton, Alberta, Canada*

"Justin showed me how to use a ball before and after I play to keep my back and shoulder feeling loose. His techniques are easy to use and remarkably effective for alleviating muscle tension and improving my performance."
- *Mat Latos – Major League Baseball Pitcher*
  (Cincinnati Reds, San Diego Padres)

"I have come across many gadgets and various techniques to release back pain and tension from aching muscles. These TBTs are simple to do and yet the results are truly unbelievable! Justin has given me an extra tool to get me and my clients to be pain-free instantly. Thank you Justin; you are a gem!"
- *Veena Kudhail, Postural Therapist, United Kingdom*

"I used these tennis ball techniques to resolve back pain that had accumulated over thirteen years of military service and six tours in Iraq and Afghanistan. In my mid-thirties my back feels as mobile, balanced, and strong as it did ten years ago, thanks to these simple techniques."
- *Special Forces Military Officer, name withheld for security reasons*

"As a Pilates professional, I thought I was practicing the safest exercise regimen available. But after years of daily exercises I started experiencing serious pain in my foot, back, and neck. With the help of The BioMechanics Method TBTs I have successfully overcome my pain."
- *Eva Wennes, Certified Pilates Instructor, North Park, California*

"The tennis ball techniques in this book will enable you to bring back elasticity to your muscles and put you in charge of bringing your body back to a pain-free state."
- *Detlef Pöhlmann, Osteopathic Doctor, Germany*

"The BioMechanics Method Tennis Ball Techniques are invaluable for anyone wanting to reduce their pain and improve their function."
-*Douglas Stewart, PhD in Biomechanics and former Director of Research for Reebok*

"I had back, hip and severe knee pain for over a year. Then I had a stroke. I did some of the tennis ball techniques in this book every day for a few weeks after my stroke. Not only did my aches and pains go away, but I have no doubt that the tennis ball techniques helped me bounce back from my stroke as quickly as I did. What a miracle cure!"
- *Joe Allen, Retired Firefighter, Missouri*

"I had tried medications, chiropractors, and various doctors, including an orthopedic surgeon, to relieve my pain - to no avail. Since working with The BioMechanics Method TBTs I am now pain-free and have even begun new interests such as kick-boxing."
- *Desiree Bobet, San Diego, California*

Acknowledgments

I would like to take a moment to express my gratitude to all the clients I have worked with over the years who enabled me to ultimately perfect these techniques. In essence, your past aches and pains are helping millions feel better today - so from me, and them, thank you! A huge thanks also goes to Frances Sharpe for your writing, editing, and creative expertise. Your involvement in the formation of this book was invaluable. My heartfelt appreciation also goes out to Laree Draper for sharing your publishing insights and knowledge and to Christine Roman for being such a patient model. Lastly, and most importantly, I would like to thank my dog, Tui, for not stealing the tennis ball every time I get on the floor to do my TBTs, and Mary for just about everything else.

Table of Contents

Introduction

Are you one of the millions of people around the world suffering from back pain? Do you toss and turn trying to find a comfortable position to sleep in? Does your aching pain keep you from enjoying the activities you love? Does a stiff, sore back interfere with your work or social life?

You're not alone. Research shows that up to 85 percent of people will experience back pain at some point in their lives. And it can strike at any age. Did you know that back pain is the most frequent cause of activity limitation in people under the age of 45? When nagging pain doesn't go away, it restricts more than your daily activities; it can also lead to psychological distress and make you feel angry, depressed, or worthless.

It's no wonder you're desperate for a cure. But finding relief can be expensive... really expensive. Every year, people in the US alone shell out at least $50 billion on back pain. This includes visits to doctors, chiropractors, physical therapists, pain specialists, and orthopedic surgeons—as well as X-rays, MRIs, and in some cases, surgeries. Some people turn to over-the-counter pain relievers while others dole out hard-earned dollars on prescription medications. And then there are all the pricy gadgets that promise relief: ergonomic chairs, pillows, beds, braces, heating pads, ice packs, and more.

What if I told you that finding relief for your aching back doesn't have to cost an arm and a leg? That it doesn't have to take hours and hours of therapy or rehabilitation? And that it doesn't require any drugs or doctors?

What if I told you that all you need to cure your back pain is a tennis ball?

How I Discovered the Amazing Tennis Ball Back Pain Cure

I first discovered how effective a tennis ball could be for pain relief when I was a professional tennis player on the international circuit. After spending grueling hours on the court or sitting in a cramped seat on a long overseas flight, my muscles would often feel tight. Whenever my body felt achy, I would reach into my bag and grab a tennis ball to help relax and massage my muscles. At the time, all I knew was that using the balls worked. I felt better almost instantly. But it wasn't until later, after I had spent years studying the human body, that I came to understand why they worked so well.

Now, as a biomechanics specialist and expert in corrective exercise techniques, I have spent more than 20 years helping people overcome chronic aches and pains. Through the years, I have developed some remarkably simple techniques that are fast, easy, and effective. And the best thing about many of them is that they involve an extremely simple tool—a tennis ball—that costs less than $1.

I teach these techniques to health and fitness professionals around the world through an educational program called The BioMechanics Method®. As a result, my methods are used by millions of people in more than 25 countries.

Now, I'm sharing The BioMechanics Method's Tennis Ball Techniques (TBTs) with you.

I have used these techniques in my own practice with people of all ages, including athletes, celebrities, Navy SEALs, heads of industry, and everyday folks like you and me. Let me introduce you to some of the people who have used these techniques to alleviate their back pain.

Jacob, 24, professional athlete: After about half a season, the right side of Jacob's lower back started to throb, and it was affecting his performance. He went to his team trainer, but no amount of icing, heating, or traditional therapies helped relieve the pain. Then he came to me and started using the TBTs. Within a few weeks, his back pain was gone and he was back in stellar form.

Mitch, 38, Navy SEAL: As you know, a Navy SEAL has to be ready for anything that comes his way. At any moment, Mitch might be sliding on the deck of a boat, standing on hard asphalt, or running in soft sand. No matter what surface he was on, he was always in tight boots that weren't ideal for all surfaces. Consequently, he experienced foot and ankle pain that eventually led to lower back pain. Using the TBTs, Mitch was able to address the problems in his feet and ankles, which alleviated the pain in his lower back. Now he uses the tennis ball for just a few minutes a day, which has kept him pain free for the past two years.

Diana, 67, grandmother and gardener: Diana was excited about moving into a new home that had a gorgeous flower garden in the backyard. But when she bent over to unpack one of the moving boxes, she doubled over in pain. For days, she could barely move. Imaging reports from a doctor showed that she had a herniated disk. Months later, her back was still so sore that she hadn't been able to do any gardening. Then she showed up at my facility and I taught her how to do the TBTs at home on her own time. A few weeks later, she called to tell me she had spent the previous week planting new flowers and her back was feeling great.

By using The BioMechanics Method's Tennis Ball Techniques, you can eliminate your back pain too, as well as any other nagging aches and pains you might have. In this book, you'll discover just how easy it can be.

Let's get started!

Chapter 1

Why Is A Tennis Ball Such An Amazing Back Pain Cure?

Can a small fuzzy green ball that costs less than $1 really cure back pain? I know it sounds too good to be true, but it's a fact. A simple tennis ball can be far more effective in relieving back pain than the expensive gadgets advertised on TV, prescriptions with their many side effects, and even surgery and other costly medical procedures. The BioMechanics Method's Tennis Ball Techniques can even do more for your aching back than stretching or spending hours at the gym doing exercises to strengthen your abdominals.

What makes The BioMechanics Method's Tennis Ball Techniques so great? Simply put, they work. To help you understand how and why they work, let me explain the most common underlying causes of back pain. Most likely, your aching back is due to one of two things:

- Muscles not working correctly *(muscular compensations)*
- Bones being out of alignment *(skeletal compensations)*

Let's take a look at each of these problems.

Muscular Compensations

Every muscle in your body has a particular job, and like most jobs in life, this often consists of a variety of tasks. For example, your glutes are in charge of helping you sit down and stand up. When you sit down, your glutes slow your hips as you lower your body so you don't go crashing to the floor. And when you want to get up, it is your glutes that provide the power to help you stand up. Your glutes also provide stability for your legs and spine while you walk.

But since we typically sit most of the day—driving to the office, hunching over our computers at work, and parking our butts on the couch to watch TV—our glutes don't have to do much. The driver's seat, office chair, and couch are doing most of the work for us. As a result, the glutes basically start sleeping on the job, and lots of smaller muscles in the butt—including one called the piriformis—take over whenever you try to stand up or sit down. When the piriformis has to pick up the slack for the glutes, it can become inflamed. That puts pressure on the sciatic nerve, which just happens to run under, over, and through the piriformis. End result? Painful sciatica.

Here's another example of how those weak glutes can be a problem for your back. When you stand up and your glutes can no longer provide a stable foundation for your spine, your body has to recruit the muscles in your lower back to keep you upright. Because your lower back is working overtime to make up for your glutes, it becomes sore and irritated. And that adds up to lower back pain.

The bottom line is that when certain muscles become weak, others have to help out. These other muscles aren't designed to handle the additional work, so they can become inflamed, which puts pressure on your nerves. It is this pressure that causes the pain in your back... not to mention in your neck, shoulders, hips, knees, and feet.

Skeletal Compensations

Have you ever sprained an ankle? If so, you probably limped around for a few days to avoid placing too much weight on it. Adjusting your movement in this manner to prevent pain in your ankle forces the rest of your body to work harder. Even in this short amount of time, compensations like these can spell trouble for the muscles and joints all the way from your ankle to your knees, hips, and back.

It takes only about 10,000 repetitions of a movement to create a new compensation habit. So when you favor an ankle, or a knee, hip, or shoulder, it can place a strain on the muscles and joints in the rest of your body very quickly. Ten thousand repetitions may seem like a lot, but you can easily rack that up in a day or two.

When this happens, your joints and bones may actually shift into the position your body thinks you want them to be in. And when your joints and bones are out of alignment, it can also put pressure on nerves, which can cause searing pain.

Skeletal compensations can also occur as a result of sitting at your computer for hours at a time. Your spine rounds forward so you can place your hands on the keyboard. Over time, this can lead to structural changes in the spine that keep you from being able to straighten your upper back when you stand up. When this occurs, your lower back has to overarch to pull you upright. This strains those hard-working muscles and puts pressure on the nerves in your lower back.

Many other everyday habits put you at risk for skeletal compensations, including:

- Carrying a purse on one side of your body
- Holding a baby or toddler on one side of your body
- Habitually carrying a briefcase with the same hand
- Wearing high-heeled shoes
- Tilting your head to one side while talking on the phone
- Walking the dog with the leash in the same hand

Whether your body develops skeletal or muscular compensations, the end result is the same; your muscles have to work harder and sometimes in ways they weren't designed to work. And that leads to pain.

Quick Compensation Test

Here's an easy way to understand how both muscular and skeletal compensations work. Fold your arms together in front of your chest. Now cross them the other way with the opposite arm on top. It feels weird for most of you, doesn't it? That's because your muscles and joints have compensated so there's only one way it feels comfortable.

Why Stretching and Strength Training May Make Back Pain Worse

Many people think that simply stretching muscles can get rid of back pain. Contrary to popular belief, stretching doesn't eradicate the problem. In fact, it can make the problem worse. If your muscles are tight, they are tight for a reason; they are responding to protect something, acting as a sort of splint for a perceived injury or an inflamed joint. When you stretch a sore muscle, it releases that muscle and may temporarily alleviate the pain. But in doing so, you also take away your body's perceived protection and stability. When you stop stretching and start moving again, the muscle almost immediately tightens back up in order to resume splinting a body part or securing a misaligned joint.

Similarly, doing exercises to strengthen your core or abdominals isn't the answer to back pain. When either your muscles or joints are out of alignment, or the little muscles of your core are doing the jobs of the big ones, core training only adds more stress to your system. Basically, by doing strength training exercises for your midsection when your body is not working correctly, you're training your body to get better at being out of alignment, which only adds to your back problems.

How The Tennis Ball Techniques Address the Underlying Causes of Back Pain

The BioMechanics Method's Tennis Ball Techniques (TBTs) can alleviate your back pain whether it is caused by muscular or skeletal compensations. In particular, they can:

- Take pressure off overworked muscles.
- Enable muscles that have gone to sleep to get back into action and start doing their job.
- Soothe irritated, inflamed muscles.
- Encourage muscles to rejuvenate and regenerate so joints and bones can return to their proper positions.

The way it works is simple; you use the tennis ball as a tool for self-massage. The use of self-massage for pain relief isn't exactly a new concept. For approximately 5,000 years, people around the world have been using some form of massage to promote health, relieve stress, and reduce pain.

Massage is thought to have originated around 2,500 to 3,000 B.C., as documented in early Chinese medical texts and in ancient Egyptian tomb paintings. Massage also has roots in traditional Indian medicine dating as far back as 1,500 B.C. The ancient Greeks and Romans also recognized the therapeutic qualities of massage and incorporated it into their daily health regimens. Even Julius Caesar used massage to help relieve pain. It wasn't until the mid-1800s that the word "massage" gained acceptance in the Western medical community.

Since then, it has become widely used around the world in all kinds of settings—from luxurious spas to high-tech hospitals. People from all walks of life take advantage of its therapeutic benefits—from weekend warriors to professional athletes, from everyday people to the President of the United States. Unsealed medical records reveal that President John F. Kennedy used massage techniques to help alleviate the unbearable foot, knee, and back pain he suffered during his career.

One of the main reasons massage has become so popular is simple: it works. We have long known it takes our aches and pains away, but thanks to new medical research, we now understand exactly how it does so. Here are just a few of the many ways massage eases pain:

- *Increases circulation:* enables oxygen and other nutrients to reach vital muscles, tissues, and organs, which helps them function better and prevents soreness
- *Increases joint flexibility:* prepares the joints for the greater range of movement and increased force

that accompanies more dynamic activities, such as exercising or playing sports, to reduce the risk of injury to muscles and joints

- *Reduces scar tissue and adhesions:* improves the elasticity of muscles and other soft tissues so your body doesn't get 'stuck' when you try to move

- *Eliminates stored tension in muscles:* allows muscles to relax and enables you to recover faster so you won't create compensations when you have sore muscles

- *Releases endorphins:* floods the body with these neurotransmitters that act as natural painkillers and help you relax, sleep better, and recover faster

- *Reduces inflammation:* helps regulate production of compounds called cytokines, which play a role in inflammation and may be involved with pain

- *Stimulates muscle repair:* increases activity in mitochondria, which are the powerhouses in cells involved in cell repair; promotes better recovery for both joints and muscles; and promotes muscle growth.

The Problem With Traditional Massage

If massage is so effective, why don't I just recommend that you head to the nearest massage therapist to cure your back pain? I'll tell you why. After helping so many people resolve their pain issues over the past 20-plus years, I have discovered that sometimes, people who give massages are not always well-qualified massage therapists and simply don't know what they're doing. In addition, a lot of individuals have issues with massage.

Take my client Sarah, for example. She told me she doesn't like having someone she doesn't know touch her. Another client, Janine, said getting a massage hurts too much and she wakes up the next day feeling like she got run over by a truck. Janine's husband, Ed, on the other hand, gets frustrated if a massage therapist doesn't rough him up by digging their elbows and fists deep into his muscles. Yet another client, Maria, confided that she hates having to take her clothes off, and worries that the massage therapist might touch her inappropriately.

Whether these fears, dislikes, and concerns are unfounded doesn't matter. The end result is that many people can't relax during a massage. If something hurts too much or you're on edge, your nervous system sees it as a potential threat and tightens up. And if you can't relax, it prevents you from getting the full benefits of massage.

Then there are the people like Martin, a busy executive who doesn't have time to go to a spa and get an hour-long massage. One young man named Ben, who I helped overcome back pain, complained about how expensive massages are.

He's right. One study put the national average cost of a one-hour massage at $76, but in some regions of the country that figure is much higher. And that's just for *one* massage. To maintain the benefits, it's best to do it on a regular basis, which means the cost adds up quickly. If you're too busy to fit a massage into your schedule or you're unable to afford it, then you aren't going to get the long-term benefits.

What about all those nifty massage gadgets? They can be costly too. Hand-held massage tools can cost upwards of $100 and massage chairs can cost as much as $10,000! One of my clients, Ruth, was very excited when her husband came home one day with a massage chair. But she soon discovered that even the lowest pressure setting was much too strong for her. The day after she used it, she woke up with bruises all over her back. She gave the chair one more try, but had the same result and hasn't used it since. She's still upset that they wasted so much money on it.

Why a Tennis Ball is the Ideal Self-Massage Tool

When you use the TBTs, you get all the benefits of massage without any of the drawbacks, which makes a tennis ball the ultimate tool for self-massage. Here's why you'll love it.

- *Get results immediately.* Within mere moments, the tension in your back—and the rest of your body—will release, and you'll feel fantastic.

- *See long-term benefits.* When you're back isn't so sore, you'll feel less stressed, you'll sleep better, you'll feel more energetic, and you'll move more effortlessly. This can help motivate you to engage in the physical activities that will boost your overall health and well-being. Whether you want to lose weight, get stronger, or excel at sports, the exercises in this book can help prepare your body to enable you to achieve these goals.

- *Enjoy better moods.* Back pain puts you in a bad mood, and a bad mood is associated with bad posture. On the other hand, good posture is associated with better moods, so when you're able to stand up straighter, you'll feel better too. The exercises in this book alleviate pain, which is one of the quickest ways to brighten your mood.

- *It puts you in charge of your pain relief.* You no longer have to rely on someone else to soothe your pain.

- *You don't have to get undressed or have some stranger rub your naked skin.* This reduces any anxiety you might have about massage and helps you relax, which helps you get the maximum benefit possible.

- *You are in complete control of the pressure.* This means that people like Janine, who like a light touch, can use an older, squishier tennis ball for a more gentle massage. People like her husband Ed can use a firmer new tennis ball for stronger pressure. (People who like it really firm can always switch to a baseball or golf ball.)

- *You can do it in private.* Use your tennis ball at home, in your office, in your hotel room, or even in your car—just keep your eyes on the road!

- *You can do it in public.* Take your tennis ball to the gym, the park, or the airport for a quick massage.

- *Do it any time of the day.* You don't have to schedule an appointment or stress about doing your tennis ball massage at a specific time of day. And you won't get sweaty doing the exercises so you can do it whenever it's most convenient for you: during your lunch break at work, while watching TV in the evening, or while waiting for your kids to finish soccer practice. Plus you can break up your routine throughout the day. Do a few minutes here and there whenever you get the chance. It offers you total flexibility as to when, where, and how you do it.

- *Greater results.* When you follow through with anything, you get better results. And because you can do this anytime or anywhere, you are far more likely to actually do it.

- *It doesn't require a lot of space.* Forget about bulky massage tables or other large equipment. Depending on which exercises you do, all you need is enough room to lie on the floor with your knees bent, sit in a chair, or stand up straight. And storage is a snap. Just toss your tennis ball into a drawer or closet when you aren't using it.

- *Take it anywhere.* A tennis ball is light (about 2 ounces) and compact (just over 2.5" in diameter), which means it will fit in handbags, briefcases, or backpacks for easy travel.

- *It's cheap.* Tennis balls are very inexpensive and easily obtainable. You can get them from most sporting goods retailers. You can even borrow one from your dog in a pinch!

- *It's quick.* You only need a few minutes a day to get relief. The exercises in this book take only 1-3 minutes each. Most people choose a few exercises and do about 10-15 minutes daily for lasting benefits.
- *It's easy to master.* There are no complicated moves or instructions to remember and no awkward positions to get into. Just follow the simple exercises in this book and start feeling better fast!

Can the Tennis Ball Techniques Help Relieve My Unique Pain?

In my line of work, I meet all kinds of people, and I understand that everybody—and *every body*—is unique. Each and every person has individual pain issues, and every body responds differently to treatment. That's why I love showing my clients how to use the TBTs. They alleviate pain from:

- Lower back problems
- Upper back problems
- Sciatica
- Disc issues
- Structural spine issues

It doesn't matter if you hurt your back in a car accident, injured yourself playing sports, or if you're just sore from everyday activities or too much sitting on the couch. The TBTs can help you rid yourself of that pain so you can get back to doing the things you love in life. Even better, because the exercises in this book target muscle tension in numerous areas of the body, they can also help you relieve other types of pain, including:

- Foot and ankle problems, such as plantar fasciitis
- Achilles tendonitis
- Knee pain, such as patella femoral syndrome and chondromalacia patella
- Calf pain
- Hip and groin pain, such as bursitis
- Sacro-iliac joint pain
- Buttocks and hamstring pain
- Shoulder pain, such as rotator cuff problems
- Carpal tunnel syndrome
- Tennis and golfer's elbow
- Neck and jaw pain
- Tension headaches

The TBTs in this book can also provide relief for the pain associated with chronic conditions, such as:

- Arthritis
- Fibromyalgia
- Neuropathy

- Irritable bowel syndrome
- Asthma
- Chronic fatigue
- Stress

Look at my patient, Ann, for example. Ann was in her late 50s and looking forward to retirement when she started experiencing debilitating pain in her back and numbness in her legs. She went to doctor after doctor, but her symptoms just kept getting worse, and she eventually lost about 90 percent of the feeling in her legs. The pain in her back was so bad that it hurt to sit down, it hurt to stand, and it was impossible to sleep through the night without being awakened by the pain. Then she got a devastating diagnosis: her doctor told her she had multiple sclerosis and that she would end up in a wheelchair. That's when Ann came to see me.

I showed her how to do the TBTs in this book, encouraging her to do them for a few minutes every day. Within three weeks, Ann's back pain was gone. After about three months, she had regained the feeling in her legs, and she felt well enough to start hiking again. She called to tell me she had gone back to the doctor who had given her the diagnosis and that, after reexamining her, he told her she *didn't* have MS.

Ann had been misdiagnosed. All she had were a number of muscular and skeletal compensations that were causing the pain and numbness. The TBTs helped her alleviate those problems.

How is Ann doing today? I know she's great because she hasn't been in to see me. I taught her how to do the exercises herself so she doesn't have to keep coming in for an appointment. I don't want my clients to be clients for life. I want to help them learn how to do these simple exercises themselves. And that's why I'm sharing these remarkable techniques with you. I want to help you avoid having to see health professionals for your back pain on a never-ending basis. I want to put you in control of your own body.

Are you ready to say good-bye to back pain and hello to the freedom of movement you used to enjoy? In the following chapter, you'll gain a better understanding of what's happening in your body, how it contributes to back pain, and how the TBTs can help you quickly eliminate that pain and keep it away for good.

Chapter 2

Why You Should Stop Blaming Your Back For Your Back Pain

As you saw in Chapter 1, your aching back may be due to other factors, so stop blaming it! The real culprit behind your back pain may be lurking somewhere else in your body. Think of your body like a major corporation with thousands of employees. All your employees work in specific departments and have specific jobs. But when any one of your body's employees takes a sick day, goes on vacation, or just goes to sleep on the job, other workers have to pitch in to get the job done. And that can stretch them beyond their capabilities and cause them stress and strain, in addition to distracting them from their own job. When some employees are doing double duty, it leads to inefficiencies, not only in that area, but also in other parts of the body.

To help you gain a better understanding of what's really causing your back to ache, let's meet some of your body's most prized employees and take a look at their job descriptions and what happens when they're overworked.

Bones: Your Body's Skeleton Crew

At birth, you have about 300 bones in your body. As you grow, some of these bones, including those in the head, pelvis, and sacrum, fuse together. By the time you reach adulthood, your skeleton has approximately 206 bones.

Job description: Your bones provide the internal framework for your body, giving it shape and providing support. They also protect your internal organs and nerves, and play a vital role in helping your muscles enable you to move. When it comes to moving your back, the spine is in charge. Otherwise known as the backbone, the spine is comprised of a collection of bones that runs from your head to your tailbone. Highly mobile, the spine is what allows you to bend, arch, and rotate your back.

When things go wrong: When other parts of your body fail to do their job, your bones have to work harder, which ultimately results in joint pain. When your joints hurt you tend to compensate by changing your gait, altering the way you stand or sit, and babying the sore joint. As you saw in Chapter 1, this can lead to back pain.

Ligaments: The Bone Connectors

The word ligament comes from the Latin word "ligare," which means "to bind or tie," and that's exactly what your ligaments do. These tough bands of tissue bind bones together at a joint. For example, they connect the thigh bones to the lower leg bones. There are also ligaments that support the internal organs—including the liver, uterus, bladder, and diaphragm—and help keep them in place.

Job description: Ligaments provide stability to joints and prevent excessive movement to prevent injury. In your spine, ligaments are attached to all the bones to allow them to move within a safe range. For example, when you twist your back, the ligaments' job is to keep your spine from rotating too far, which could cause injury.

When things go wrong: When ligaments are overstretched, they can sprain or tear, which may result in destabilization of the joint. This forces you to create harmful compensations that can lead to back pain.

Muscles: The Movers and Shakers

When you want to get moving, you have to recruit your muscles. But not all muscles are created equal. In your body, there are three types of muscles:

- *Smooth muscles:* These regulate unconscious movement in the body, such as digesting food or breathing.
- *Cardiac muscles:* These keep your heart beating.
- *Skeletal muscles:* These are typically attached to the bones and are under your conscious control. The most common type of muscle in the body, there are more than 650 skeletal muscles at your beck and call.

Job description: Your skeletal muscles are responsible for creating movement by either contracting or lengthening. It is their job to spring into action every time you move, whether you want to walk, run, jump, reach, pull, push, bend, or twist.

When things go wrong: As you saw in Chapter 1, muscles that are overworked can become inflamed and place pressure on nerves that cause back pain flare-up.

Tendons: The Muscle-Bone Middlemen

Tendons are tough yet flexible connective tissues that act like middlemen between your muscles and your bones.

A tendon is formed where the fibers come together at either end of a muscle, similar to the way a bouquet of roses is gathered at the bottom. This tapering of the muscle is what enables it to attach, via the tendon, to the appropriate site on the bone. The Achilles tendon, which attaches the calf muscle to the heel, is the best-known of these sinewy tissues, but you have tendons throughout your body, including your back.

Job description: Your tendons' primary job is to connect muscle to bone, but they also work with the muscles and bones to help you move. As your muscles contract, the tendons pull on the bones to create the movement. Tendons must be rigid enough, yet also flexible enough, to make sure they don't detach from the bone.

When things go wrong: Excessive wear and tear on a tendon can cause it to become inflamed, a condition referred to as tendonitis. Tendonitis, which becomes more common with age, can lead to compensations and problems with your back.

Fascia: The Systems Integrator

Every company needs employees that help integrate all the various departments of the firm so that everybody understands the company's goals and is heading in the same direction. In your body, that job belongs to fascia, a three-dimensional web of connective tissue that runs uninterrupted from the top of the head to the tips of the toes. Fascia holds together all the bones, ligaments, muscles, and tendons in your body. It also weaves its way through and around nearly every tissue in the body, including veins, arteries, organs, and nerves.

Job description: Fascia basically integrates all the systems in your body to enable them to move together as a cohesive unit. When fascia is healthy, it allows you to move without pain.

When things go wrong: When structures of the body are either out of alignment or not working correctly, the entire system is affected, including the fascia. Unhealthy fascia is prone to develop painful issues, such as excessive tightness, nodules, adhesions, and inflexibility. This may occur anywhere in the body and can be felt in the back.

Posture: Your Body's Balance Sheet

How can you tell if your body's employees are doing their job to the best of their abilities, or if they are slacking off on company time? All you have to do is take a look at your posture. The same way a company's balance sheet provides an immediate glimpse into its state of affairs, your posture offers a clear picture of the health of your musculoskeletal system. When all your body's workers are doing their job correctly, you stand upright with shoulders back, chin level, and eyes forward. But when even a single employee is turning in a less-than-stellar performance, your posture suffers. Some of the many telltale signs of poor posture include:

- slumping
- shoulders hunched forward
- back rounded
- hip hiked to one side
- shoulder drooped on one side
- knock knees
- flat feet
- head pitched forward

Don't blame yourself for your poor posture. Our modern environment contributes greatly to the problem. Think about it; our human ancestors had to walk, run, climb, and jump on a regular basis. Whatever they wanted to accomplish, they had to move their bodies to do it. Today, our bodies are still designed for that kind of physical activity, but we rarely use them that way. Instead, we spend more time sitting, driving, and staring at screens than we do being physically active. And even when we are walking, we are often looking down while we text or email, or cocking our heads to the side while talking on our cell phones. Our society's relentless quest for convenience has come at a high price; our bodies have gotten out of balance and become deconditioned.

Today, our muscles, tendons, and fascia spend most of their time on vacation. But then we expect them to perform at top level when we participate in strenuous activities like playing sports, going to the gym, or hiking. It's as if a company's assembly line produces one product per day and then once a week, once a month, or once in a blue moon, the boss rushes in and announces that it has to churn out 100 in a single hour.

Imagine how overloaded you would feel as an employee, how much more likely you would be to make mistakes, or just throw your hands in the air and give up. On an assembly line, when one person doesn't do his job, it causes a logjam that affects everyone else down the line. The same goes for our bodies.

The Gravity Factor

When things go haywire in the body, it causes grave problems—or rather, gravity problems. You remember learning about gravity in school; it's what keeps us from floating off into space. Gravity is constantly pulling every part of our bodies downward, and we have to work to stay upright or we will end up in a heap on the floor. We stay upright thanks to our muscles, tendons, fascia, ligaments, and bones working together.

But as you have seen, our muscles, tendons, and fascia have forgotten, in large part, how to do their jobs. If these employees are out to lunch, the remaining key players have to pitch in to keep us from falling down. Consequently, the job of working against gravity eventually falls to our ligaments and bones, which dutifully take over, locking the joints together to maintain stability. This results in joint pain.

Gravity can take a toll on our bodies in other ways as well. As it pulls and pulls, it may cause parts of your body to literally collapse. For example, the arches in your feet may fall, giving you flat feet. But your problem doesn't stop at your feet. Look at the chain of events that occurs when your arches collapse:

- your ankles roll inward;
- your knees knock;
- the top of your leg shifts to the back;
- your pelvis tips up on your backside, making your lower back overarch;
- your pelvis pitches downward in front so your abs pooch out;
- your upper back rounds;
- your neck juts forward;
- you have to tilt your head up to look forward.

It's not a pretty picture. And it doesn't always start with the feet. Any one of these problems can set off a chain reaction throughout the body.

Did You Know?

Your head weighs about 8 pounds, which is what your spine and muscles are designed to support. But for every inch your head juts forward, it doubles the weight your body has to bear. So if your neck is pitched just 2" forward, it's like having to carry around 32 pounds on top of your neck instead of 8 pounds. That puts stress on your spine and back muscles, causing pain.

Why Your Back Bears the Brunt of the Pain

If you were experiencing all the bodily malfunctions that come as a result of those fallen arches in the earlier example, you would probably expect to be in pain from head to toe. But that isn't necessarily the case. You could have all these things going wrong in your body but only feel soreness in—you guessed it—your back. How can that be? Take a look at some of the reasons why your back is the area that is most likely to feel the pain.

- Your back muscles are some of the biggest muscles in your body, so when other muscles don't do their job, the back muscles often take over, which causes stress, strain, and inflammation.
- Your back is where you have the highest concentration of nerves, and more nerve endings means more pain receptors.
- Your back is also where the largest nerves in the body can be found and *big* nerves equal *big* pain receptors.

When gravity is taking its toll and your whole body is collapsing, the big muscles in your back put a lot of stress on those nerves. Essentially your back is having a nervous breakdown, literally! This is why you may feel pain more sharply in your back, even when the root of the problem lies elsewhere in your body, and why you can't just focus on treating your back to alleviate back pain.

Why You Have to Target More Than Just Your Aching Back

Because back pain may be a symptom of dysfunction throughout the body, you can't just massage the painful area on your back and expect to get relief. If that's all you do, the pain will keep coming back. I guarantee it. To get lasting relief, you have to address your whole body. And the TBTs can help you do this.

In just a few minutes a day you can loosen muscles and awaken sleeping muscles, soothe irritated tendons and ligaments, and release knots and adhesions in the fascia—all of which will help realign bones. When muscles are working properly, it takes stress off the tendons. When your bones are in better alignment, they are less likely to press on nerves, overstretch ligaments, and cause inflammation in your tissues. By reconditioning your body with the exercises in this book, you will ultimately take pressure off those nerves in your back, which will finally eliminate the pain.

When your bones, muscles, ligaments, tendons, and fascia are working the way they are intended to work, you will experience the joy of pain-free movement. No more waking up feeling creaky and stiff, no more shifting endlessly in your chair to avoid the shooting pain down your leg, no more dreading social occasions where you have to stand around for hours, and no more avoiding the activities you love.

When all the employees in your company—that is, your body—are performing at peak capacity, you'll see it in your posture. You'll stand up straighter, breathe more freely, and you'll actually be taller. But even more important, you'll have a lot less pain and a lot more fun in your life.

Chapter 3

Getting The Most Out Of The BioMechanics Method Tennis Ball Techniques

As you have seen, you can't just focus on your back if you want to alleviate back pain. Because your whole body is interconnected you need to address the whole system. That's exactly what The BioMechanics Method's Tennis Ball Techniques (TBTs) do. When I first talk to my clients about the TBTs, they inevitably have questions. You probably do too. To help you get the most out of the tennis ball techniques in the next chapter, I've put together the following Q&A, featuring the most common questions I get from my clients. You will find the answers to any questions you may have here.

Where do I begin?

There are three things you need to do prior to getting your tennis ball out in order to get the most out of your TBTs.

1. *Become aware of the activities you typically engage in during the week and on the weekends.* For example, do you spend most of the time sitting at your desk, standing at a counter, driving your kids around, or playing sports? Do you sit at your computer all week then expect to be a sporting weekend warrior? Do you work out every day? Do you have a long commute to and from work? Do you sit during lunch or go for a walk? Are your weekend activities different than your weekday activities? Are your weekend activities more sedentary—like going to the movies or going out to dinner—or more active—like going for a hike or a bike ride? Knowing your activities will help you zero in on the TBTs that are best for you.

2. *Become aware of your pain.* You may think you are already acutely aware that your back hurts, but I want you to really get in touch with the aches

and pains all over your body. Make a mental note, or even better, get a notepad to keep track of your pain for a week on a day-to-day or even hour-by-hour basis, if necessary. Determine exactly where the pain in your back is located: on your lower right side, closer to your tailbone, in your mid-upper back, or more on top of your butt and hips. Also track and note pain in other parts of your body. Notice if your pain is worse during the week or on weekends, in the morning or in the evening, after strenuous activity or after sitting at your desk or in the car, after a night out wearing high heels or after going barefoot at home. The point is to become conscious of when and where you feel pain.

3. *Take note of any past injuries or surgeries.* These can lead to scar tissue and adhesions that affect muscles and fascia. For example, let's say you sprained your ankle a few years ago. The muscles and fascia around the ankle would have tightened to help keep the joint from moving while it healed. As a result of this tightness, your body may have compensated to adjust for the lack of mobility in your ankle. So now you may have residual back pain because of the old sprain. Although

your ankle may not hurt anymore, it may be responsible for your back pain.

Similarly, surgical scars cause tightness that can lead to compensations and ultimately, back pain. You may be surprised to learn that many of my female clients with back pain have had a hysterectomy or C-section that cut through the abdominal wall. The resulting scar tissue inhibits the ab muscles and fascia from working optimally, which can lead to problems with the spine. So even though you have completely recovered from your procedure, you may still be feeling the effects.

How do I know which TBTs are best for me?

Use the information you have gathered on your daily activities, pain, and injuries and/or surgeries to guide you to the techniques that will be most helpful to you.

1. *Be guided by your daily activities.* For example, if you spend a lot of time sitting down, then the muscles in your hips, butt, and lower and upper back are probably unhealthy. Use a tennis ball to recondition the muscles in these areas. If you stand a lot, use a tennis ball to release tension in your feet and calf muscles, as well as the muscles around your spine that are helping to keep your

torso upright. If you engage in sporting activities on the weekend, use the tennis ball techniques to release those muscles and fascia that have been affected by your activities. For example, if you play tennis, or golf, or swim, then focus on using a tennis ball to release the muscles around the shoulders in addition to your feet, hips, and back. If you go for a hike or jog, use the tennis ball to loosen the muscles of your feet, calves, legs, hips, and lower back. If you go out on a Saturday night and wear high heels, then loosen up your feet, calf, and back muscles when you get home or in the morning, to help relieve tension from the calves and low back.

2. *Be guided by your pain.* Refer to your list of painful areas to decide which exercises to do. For example, if you've been gardening or housecleaning and your upper back hurts at the end of the day, choose the TBTs that target that area. If you've spent the day walking, sightseeing, or standing around while your kids play soccer, do the TBTs for your legs and feet. Don't do the same TBTs all the time. Vary them to address the specific areas of your body that are causing you problems. For example, if you go hiking on uneven trails and

notice the next day that the muscles on the out-side of your lower leg are really sore, make sure to add the TBTs for the outside of the leg.

3. *Be guided by your injuries and/or surgeries.* Refer to your list of past injuries and/or surgeries and zero in on those areas. For example, if you've had a knee or hip replacement, use a tennis ball on the muscles near those joints to break up any scar tissue or muscle restrictions that may have formed as a result of the surgery. This will help get that area to move more freely.

If, after reviewing your activities, pain, and injuries and/or surgeries, you are still having trouble identify-ing which TBTs are best for you, refer to the guide for each technique and/or the handy guide at the end of the following chapter to direct you to the best exercises for your needs.

Do The BioMechanics Method's Tennis Ball Techniques hurt?

You can initially expect to feel some discomfort when you use them. This is because you are pushing on mus-cles and fascia that are tight and irritated and that are, in turn, pressing on nerves. However, rest assured that the experience should not produce severe pain. Always listen to your own body. If it feels too painful, apply less pressure or try an older, softer tennis ball. Ideally, you should be able to relax enough to keep sustained pressure on sore areas.

You may notice that some areas of your body produce more pain than others. This may be because the muscles in those areas are tighter or it may simply be due to the fact that there are more nerves in these particular areas. In either case, you may need to apply lighter pressure to these areas, compared to other parts of your body.

Should the discomfort dissipate as I do the TBTs?

Yes, as you do the exercises, you should begin to feel some relief in sore areas. If the pain doesn't diminish, ease up or move the tennis ball to another spot nearby that isn't quite so angry. After loosening up the surrounding tissues, go back to the original spot and see if it is more tolerable. When you find a spot that is very tender, it's important that you don't stick it out and try to work through the discomfort. A very sore muscle is likely to go into protection mode and tighten up even more, which won't give you the benefits you want.

How will I know that I'm using the tennis ball in the right spot?

If you feel some discomfort, you're probably in the right spot. If you don't feel anything, keep moving the tennis ball around an area until you feel some discomfort. That's the spot that needs attention. You can also refer to the TBT placement guides in the next chapter for assistance.

Should I just focus on that one particular spot?

No. Although it is a good idea to spend a little more time with the tennis ball on spots that cause the most discomfort, it is better to explore the surrounding area as well. As you know, the body is interconnected, so this will promote healing to the entire affected area—not just one spot.

Should I be actively rolling around on the ball?

No, it is not a good idea to roll around on the ball. If you try to maneuver your body back and forth or side to side on the ball, your muscles have to spring into action to stabilize your body. This causes your muscles to tighten, which is counterproductive. The best approach is to place the tennis ball in one spot, wait for the soreness to release (see chapter 4 for recommendations on how long to hold the tennis ball in place), then move the ball to a new spot. Additionally, if you roll around on the ball you may accidentally roll directly over a nerve, which can hurt both you and the nerve.

Should I really dig in and do it as hard as possible to make improvements faster?

No. I recommend you take a more gentle approach. Remember, the tightness in your body didn't get there overnight, and you won't get it out overnight. If you push too hard with the tennis ball your body may interpret the pain as potential harm and tighten up. This can prevent your body from relaxing and releasing tension and gaining the maximum benefits from the TBTs.

What should I do if using the tennis ball on a certain area is just too painful?

As mentioned before, if this is the case, ease up. Use a softer ball, such as an older tennis ball, or angle your body differently on the ball to alleviate the discomfort. When the area eventually starts to loosen up, you can reintroduce a newer tennis ball or angle your body more directly on the spot. As always, let your body be the guide. Information on how to make each TBT easier or less uncomfortable is included in the next chapter.

What if I have pain in a particular area, but I don't feel anything when I put a tennis ball there?

If there is an area of your body that is extremely tight, and it has been for years, you may not feel any discomfort or pressure when you first place a tennis ball there. This is likely because the muscles and fascia are so tight they won't release even a little bit in order for the ball to get through to the nerves. If you stay on the spot for a minute or two, the muscles will eventually release and you will start to feel the pressure.

How do I know when I'm ready to progress to a harder tennis ball?

When massaging with the ball no longer produces any discomfort, it's time to try a harder tennis ball. Eventually, you may want to progress to a baseball or similar hard ball, such as a lacrosse or cricket ball.

Can I do more than one TBT to work several areas at once so I can save time?

No, it is best to concentrate on one general area at a time. Many of my clients tell me that they want to save time by using multiple tennis balls on their hips, back, and neck at the same time. But doing so is ultimately inefficient because you have to think about too many things, balance yourself awkwardly, or constantly reposition balls; and you can't relax. Doing more than one TBT at a time doesn't allow you to get the benefits you need.

Does it matter what kind of mood I'm in when I do the TBTs?

As you have seen, it is important for your muscles to relax to get the most out of the exercises. Therefore, it is best to be in a relaxed frame of mind when you do the exercises. If you're stressed because you just spent an hour in traffic, the TBTs will help you chill out. However, if the kids are running around screaming while you are doing your exercises, your body goes into protective mode and won't settle down enough to enable your muscles to relax.

Should I do the TBTs before or after activity/exercise?

It's up to you. There are good arguments for both. Doing them before activity will help loosen up your muscles and get your body in better alignment, so you can perform the activity with less stress to your skeletal system. Doing them after will help your muscles recover faster and get your body back in alignment if you have "tweaked" anything. If you have time, do the TBTs both before and after activities. If not, try both options and see which one works best for you.

Should I do the TBTs in a particular order?

It is recommended that you start with the ones that target the bigger muscles, like your butt, hips, legs, and back. This will bring blood supply to these muscles, which will help warm up your entire body and enable it to relax, so that you get more benefit when you do the exercises on the smaller muscles.

Is it okay to do the TBTs immediately following a sprain or injury?

In some cases, you may need to wait a few days until an acute injury, such as an ankle sprain, has healed or the initial inflammation has subsided. Use ice for up to three days after an injury for about 20 minutes each day to help reduce inflammation in the joint. After that, you can start helping the muscles around the area heal with the TBTs. For other issues—which may be chronic or acute—such as throwing your back out, pulling a muscle, or extreme muscle tension, you can use a tennis ball on those tight muscles to help them release and take pressure off the nerves. Also, using the TBTs after an injury can help prevent compensations and subsequent chronic pain.

Should I use heat or ice on my muscles in addition to or instead of doing the TBTs?

If an area is extremely tight and the pressure of a ball is too painful, use a heating pad on those muscles for about 20-30 minutes each day for a few days. Then try using the TBTs again to see if there is less discomfort. Ice may help numb pain and reduce inflammation to joints, but won't do much to help correct the underlying causes of your pain.

What should I wear while doing the TBTs?

It really doesn't matter what you're wearing. Whether you're in a suit in the office or sweat pants at the gym, you can get relief. If you're sitting down while using a tennis ball on your back, it doesn't even matter if you're wearing high heels—although I have to remind you that those stilettos may be contributing to your back pain when you're on your feet. You may also want to empty your pockets and remove any belts so the balls can put pressure on the right areas if you are targeting your hips or lower back.

Do I need to warm up before doing the TBTs?

It is not necessary to perform any type of warm-up routine. However, if you feel particularly sore or achy on a given day, you could take a warm shower or bath before you do the TBTs. This will help bring blood supply to your muscles and loosen them up so you can get the most benefit from the tennis balls.

Should I do the TBTs every day?

Ideally, you should spend a few minutes every day doing them. However, if you are really busy, don't beat yourself up if you miss a day. Even if you can't do the TBTs every day, don't give up. You will still gain some benefit.

Should I continue doing the TBTs even after my back pain has subsided?

After back pain has been alleviated, it is very common for people to stop doing the exercises and fall back into their old patterns and habits of movement. In some cases, this results in a flare-up of their pain. For this reason, I recommend you continue with the TBTs on a regular basis, even when your back is no longer aching. The great thing about these exercises is that even if you stop doing them and your back pain returns, you'll know exactly what to do to alleviate it. If pain resurfaces, go back to doing the TBTs every day to get relief.

Are the TBTs a short-term Band-Aid or a long-term solution?

The answer is both. They can be a quick fix in an emergency as well as a long-term solution for your back pain. When you tweak your back or strain a hamstring muscle, you can use the TBTs right away to help soothe the irritated area and promote rapid healing. When you use the exercises on a regular basis, you can get to the underlying causes of your back pain and get rid of it for good.

Why didn't my chiropractor, physical therapist, or orthopedic surgeon tell me about these kinds of exercises?

I can't say for sure, but it may be because they aren't familiar with these techniques or how beneficial they can be. Many professionals know that the body is interconnected, but they may not understand all the ways it works together because they are trained to specialize in specific areas or parts of the body only. Plus, many healthcare practitioners focus on addressing your symptoms—that is, your pain. Also, a lot of them simply don't have the time to teach you techniques to help you change the way your body functions.

It is easier for some medical professionals to recommend having surgery to fix problems caused by alignment issues, such as a herniated disc. However, this may only be a temporary solution because surgery isn't going to address the underlying muscle or skeletal imbalances that contributed to the problem in the first place. It's the same with some chiropractors, who may get your joints in alignment, but if you don't address the condition of the muscles and fascia, they will pull you back out of alignment and you'll end up with same problem. Then there is the sad fact that some professionals may not want to share this type of information with you because they won't make any money by teaching you how to help yourself get better.

So why am I being so generous? Because helping people learn how to heal their own pain using the TBTs is the best advertising I could possibly get. Every time I help someone, they go out and tell their friends, family, and coworkers how much better they feel. The resulting word-of-mouth referrals are what make me one of the most sought-after pain-relief specialists in the world.

Can I injure myself doing the TBTs?

No, if you do them correctly, you are not going to injure yourself. These exercises have been developed with safety in mind, to put you in complete control. If you feel too much pain while using the tennis ball, simply use a softer ball or apply less pressure. You are in charge, so you don't have to worry about causing additional pain.

What if I hear a popping noise in my back while doing the TBTs?

Don't worry. A popping noise usually indicates that the spine is naturally adjusting to a better position, which is a good thing. This natural "re-alignment" is better for you in the long run than continually getting adjustments from a chiropractor. Here's why. Tight muscles, fascia, and tendons are typically what pull the bones out of alignment. When you release them by using the TBTs, the bones can fall back into their correct positions naturally, and this may make a popping noise. A chiropractor mainly addresses alignment problems of the body by forcefully repositioning bones. However, tight muscles, fascia, and tendons will inevitably pull them back out.

Because your whole body is interconnected, you may notice that other areas may also pop while you do the TBTs. For example, as you do them for your back, you may find your knees or hips pop too. This is completely natural and indicates that the structures of the body are falling back into better alignment.

My arm goes to sleep when I use the tennis ball on my upper back. Why does this happen and what should I do?

In some positions, the ball may rest directly on a nerve, which can cause a temporary tingling sensation or feeling of numbness in another area. If this occurs, don't be alarmed. Simply reposition the tennis ball and feeling should return to the area.

What's the difference between using a foam roller and a tennis ball for self-massage?

A foam roller is an adequate tool for massaging big surfaces, but it is not small enough to address many of the specific muscles that contribute to back pain. Also, foam rollers are bulky and unwieldy; they certainly don't fit in a purse or briefcase. And many people find it hard to balance on them. If you're using the roller on your upper back, for example, you have to hold your neck up, which causes the muscles in your neck and upper back to tense, which diminishes the effect of the exercise. Because foam rollers are large in diameter, you also have to prop yourself up while using them, which makes it harder to relax.

A tennis ball, on the other hand, is small enough to target both large and small muscles and fascia. It is lightweight and portable, and it doesn't present any balance issues, which allows you to relax and get the most out of the exercises.

My doctor told me I should just rest my back to get rid of the pain. Are the TBTs better than rest?

The age-old advice to "rest" in order to reduce back pain is a bit inadequate. Here's why. I had a client named Todd who threw his back out. When he went to the doctor, he was advised to lie in bed for four days to get the inflammation down. Though this approach may have helped temporarily, it didn't solve the underlying issues that had led to the problem in the first place. Todd stayed in bed for the four days, then went right back to his old routines. A few months later, he threw his back out again. It was a vicious cycle. Fortunately, after the second episode, Todd came to see me and learned how to correct the underlying causes of his back pain.

Why can't I just wear orthotics or arch supports if my feet are contributing to my back pain?

As you have seen, problems with your feet can lead to a chain of compensations throughout the body that results in back pain. But foot problems may also be just a symptom of dysfunction elsewhere in the body. Wearing orthotics or arch supports to artificially support the feet may help in the short-term, but it doesn't address the underlying muscle imbalances that may have contributed to the original problems. You still need the TBTs to correct those.

My wife sees me doing my TBTs and wants to try them, though she doesn't have back pain. Is that a good idea?

It's a great idea! As a society, we're usually very reactive when it comes to our health. We wait until we have a problem, then panic and throw a lot of money at it to try to make it go away. Using the TBTs when you don't have a problem is proactive, costs very little money, and can keep your body in top working order.

Can anyone use The BioMechanics Method's Tennis Ball Techniques?

The exercises in this book are suitable for people of all ages. However, it is a good idea to check with your physician prior to starting any type of exercise routine. It is especially important to get physician approval for a child or teen who is still growing.

Are there any other special considerations I need to think about?

In general, it's always best to use common sense when applying the techniques in this book. But here are a few special considerations you may want to keep in mind. If you have any concerns about your physical condition or the TBTs, check with your physician first.

- Don't place the tennis ball on areas that are badly bruised or swollen.
- Don't use the ball on areas that are actively in spasm.
- As with any exercise, if you have severely high blood pressure, check with your doctor before doing the TBTs.
- If you are a pregnant woman in the third trimester, it is not advisable to be on the ground on your

belly or back for long periods of time, so keep TBT sessions brief.

- Don't do the TBTs if you have the flu, a high fever, or other severe ailment.

- If you have recently had abdominal surgery, such as a C-section or hysterectomy, avoid placing the tennis ball on the abdominal area until your doctor says it's okay to do so.

- If you have severe rheumatoid arthritis or osteoporosis, be very gentle in the areas that are affected.

- Don't use the tennis ball on broken bones.

- If you have varicose veins, it's okay to use the TBTs, but be gentle.

- The two bottom ribs just above your waist don't attach to the sternum, so don't apply extreme pressure in that area.

- Don't do the TBTs if you are dehydrated, especially as a result of excessive alcohol consumption.

Chapter 4

The Amazing Tennis Ball Techniques

Here are the techniques you've been waiting for! The 16 TBTs in this chapter can help address both muscular and skeletal compensations throughout your body, to alleviate pain in your back—as well as your feet and ankles, knees, hips, shoulders, wrists and hands, and neck.

The following information has been included for each TBT to help you know exactly what to expect:

- The name of the TBT and a corresponding number for easy reference
- How the exercise can relieve your pain, accompanied by a photo of the technique in action

- An anatomy graphic to help you know where to put the ball
- A guide to help you determine if that specific TBT is right for you
- Instructions on how to do the exercise
- Notations on how long and how often you should do it
- Helpful tips and/or precautions
- Ways to make the TBT harder and/or easier.

If you have any general questions before you get started, refer to Chapter 3, where you will find the answers you're looking for. Remember to start slowly and *gradually* progress to doing more exercises as your body feels better.

Important Information
The information, instruction, and techniques contained in this book are in no way intended to be a substitute for medical counsel or advice. Prior to engaging in any exercise program, including the tennis ball techniques outlined in this book, you are advised to seek medical evaluation and/or clearance from a doctor. Not all exercise programs are suitable for everyone and some programs may, in fact, result in injury. Techniques such as those depicted in this book should be carried out at a level that is comfortable for the individual engaging in the activity. You should discontinue participation in any exercise or activity that causes pain or severe discomfort. In such an event, medical consultation should immediately be obtained.

TBT #1

Tennis Ball Under Foot

This TBT helps regenerate and rejuvenate the muscles and fascia on the underside of the foot.

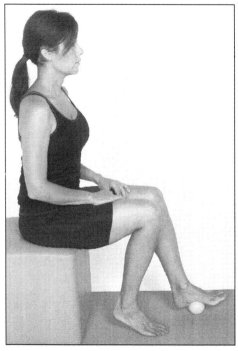

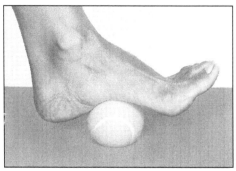

Where do I put the ball?

There are many muscles, ligaments, bones, tendons, and fascia that help shape the underside of your feet. You will be targeting a tissue that stretches along the entire bottom of your foot, called the plantar fascia, to help your feet function better and to ease your back pain.

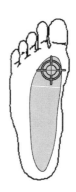

Do this TBT if you:

Stand a lot; walk a lot; run; wear shoes that don't allow your toes to spread out; have bunions or calluses on your feet; play sports on your feet; have foot and/or ankle pain, knee pain, back pain; have ever broken or sprained a toe or ankle, or had foot surgery.

How do I do it?

Roll the bottom of your foot over the tennis ball. When you find a particularly sore spot, maintain pressure on it for 5 – 10 seconds to help it release. Do each foot for 1 to 2 minutes.

Tips

Keep a tennis ball beside the couch, your favorite chair, or under your desk, so you can do this while you watch television or are on the computer. To make this TBT harder, pull your toes toward your shin and/or do it standing up, to apply more pressure to the bottom of your foot.

Precautions

Do not apply too much pressure if you use a hard ball for this TBT.

TBT #2

Tennis Ball Under Calf

This TBT will help loosen the muscles and fascia on the back of the lower leg.

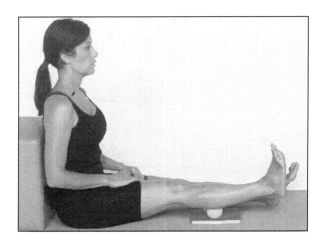

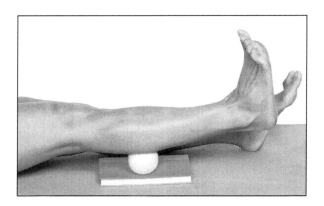

Where do I put the ball?

There are two big muscles on the back of your calf that attach to your heel via the Achilles tendon (i.e., gastrocnemius and soleus). When healthy and flexible, these muscles enable your ankles and knees to function correctly, which can thwart ankle, knee, and back pain.

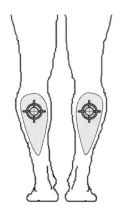

Do this TBT if you:

Stand a lot; walk a lot; run; sit a lot; wear high-heeled shoes; play sports on your feet; are overweight; have bunions and/or calluses on your feet; have foot and/or ankle pain, knee pain, back pain; have injured a knee or ankle, or had knee surgery.

How do I do it?

Sit on the floor with your back against a wall with your legs outstretched. Place a tennis ball on top of a hardcover book and lower the back of your calf to rest on top of the ball. Find a sore spot on your calf and maintain pressure on it for 5-10 seconds until it releases. Then move to the next spot. Do each leg for about 1 to 2 minutes.

Tips

This exercise is easy to do while sitting on the couch because you can place the ball on a coffee table or ottoman instead of the floor. To make it harder, pull your toes up toward your shin and/or place the other leg on top of the leg you are massaging to increase pressure to the ball.

Precautions

If you use a hard ball for this exercise (e.g., a baseball) do not apply direct pressure to the back of the knee or on the Achilles tendon itself (which is just above the back of the heel).

TBT #3

Tennis Ball Side Of Calf

This TBT helps recondition the muscles and fascia on the outside of the lower leg.

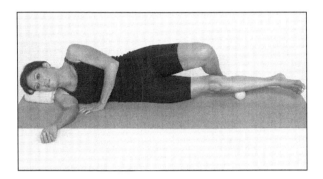

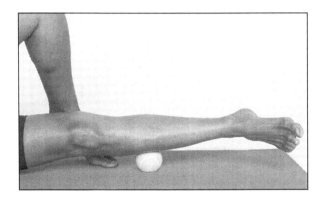

Where do I put the ball?

There are muscles on the outside of your lower leg called the peroneals. These help control the lower leg and foot when you walk. This TBT can help keep them supple and healthy, so they work well and eliminate unnecessary stress to the foot, ankle, knee, hip, and back.

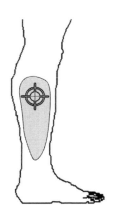

Do this TBT if you:

Stand a lot; walk a lot; run; ski; play sports that require side-to-side movements like tennis; have bunions or callouses on your feet; have pain on the outside of your foot and/or ankle; tend to wear down the outside of your shoes; or have ever sprained or broken your ankle or a little toe.

How do I do it?

Lie on your right side with your legs outstretched. Place the outside of your lower leg on top of a tennis ball. Place your left leg on top of your right leg to increase the pressure, if necessary. Find a sore spot and maintain pressure on it until it releases (5-10 seconds). Then move to the next spot. Repeat on the other leg. Do each leg for about 1 to 2 minutes.

Tips

Use a pillow to support your head when lying on your side. This will help keep your neck in line with the rest of your spine. To make this TBT easier, take the top leg off the bottom leg (see photo).

Precautions

If you use a hard ball for this exercise, do not place direct pressure just above the outside of the ankle bone (there is a tendon there).

TBT #4

Tennis Ball On Front Of Thigh

This TBT helps loosen the muscles on the front of the thigh.

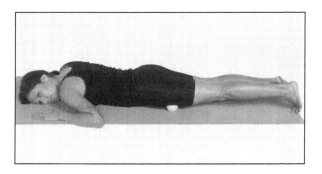

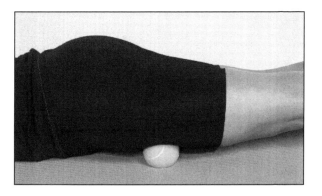

Where do I put the ball?

There are four big muscles on the front of
your thigh called your quadriceps. They
help control movement of the knee; one
even helps with movement of the pelvis.
Releasing tension from these muscles enables them to function better, which can
lessen knee, hip, and back pain.

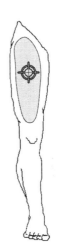

Do this TBT if you:

Sit at a computer; lean forward at work;
squat or lunge; walk a lot; jog or run; ski; play sports on
your feet; have back or knee pain; had back or knee surgery; or a knee replacement, hip surgery, or ankle surgery.

How do I do it?

Lie face down on the floor with your legs outstretched.
Place a tennis ball under the front of your right thigh.
Find a sore spot and maintain pressure on it until it releases (5-10 seconds). Then move to the next spot. Release
all the sore spots from the top of your thigh to just above
your kneecap. Make sure to do both legs. Do each for
about 1 to 2 minutes.

Tips

As with most of the exercises in this book, you can do this one while lying on the floor and watching TV or in bed (if you place the ball on top of a hardcover book to prevent it from sinking into the mattress). You can also place two or three tennis balls in a sock so you can do a larger area of the leg each time you move the balls.

Precautions

When using a hard ball for this exercise, do not place direct pressure just above the kneecap (there is a tendon there).

TBT #5

Tennis Ball On Side Of Leg

This TBT helps recondition the band of connective tissue and fascia that runs down the side of the leg.

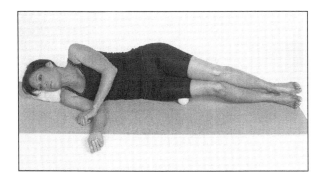

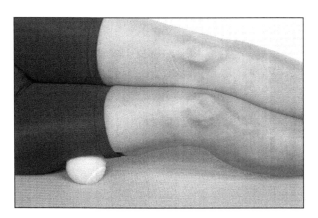

Where do I put the ball?

There is a strip of connective tissue called the iliotibial band that runs along the outside of the upper leg from the side of the hip to just below the knee. When this tissue is healthy and free from restrictions, it assists the muscles of the hips and butt to work correctly, which can decrease back, hip, and knee pain.

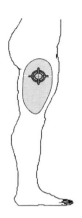

Do this TBT if you:

Stand a lot; squat or lunge; walk; run; ride a bike; ski; swim; wear high heels or walk on uneven surfaces; play sports on your feet; have back, hip, knee, or ankle pain; had knee surgery (including a knee replacement); or surgery on the back, hips, and/or ankle.

How do I do it?

Lie on the floor on your right side with your legs outstretched. Place a tennis ball under your upper leg on the outside of your right thigh. Place your left leg on top of your right leg to increase the pressure, if necessary. Find a sore spot and maintain pressure on it until it releases (5-10 seconds). Then move to the next spot. Release all the sore spots from the top of your leg to just above your kneecap. Make sure you do both legs. Do each for about 1 to 2 minutes.

Tips

If the ball slips from under your leg, set it on a rolled up towel or small pillow to hold it in place. You can also place two or three tennis balls in a sock so you can do a larger area of the leg each time you move the balls.

Precautions

When using a harder ball for this exercise, do not place direct pressure on the side of the knee or the side of the hip.

TBT #6

Tennis Ball On Inner Thigh

This TBT will help rejuvenate and recondition the muscles of the inner thigh.

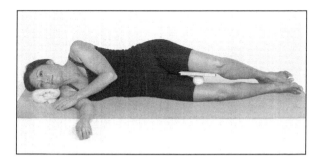

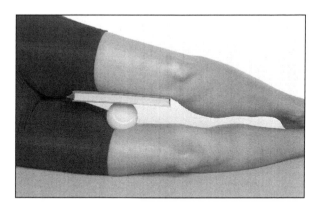

Where do I put the ball?

There are several muscles that run along the inside of the thigh called the adductor muscles. This TBT targets the adductors and the fascia of the inner thigh to help keep these tissues supple and stretchy so the leg, hips, and lower back can function correctly and feel better.

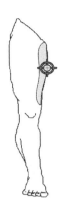

Do this TBT if you:

Stand a lot; squat or lunge; water ski; snow ski; walk; run; go up and down stairs a lot; walk on uneven surfaces; play sports on your feet where you have to move side-to-side often—like in basketball; have back, hip, or knee pain; had a knee replacement or surgery of the knee, back, hips, and/or ankle.

How do I do it?

Lie on your right side and place a tennis ball on the inner thigh of your right leg. Place a small book on top of the tennis ball and your left leg on top of the book. Find a sore spot and maintain pressure on it until it releases (5-10 seconds). Then move to the next spot. Release all the sore spots from the top of your inner thigh to just above your kneecap. Flip over and repeat on the other leg. Do each leg for about 1 to 2 minutes.

Tips

A hardcover book will produce more pressure, a paperback less pressure. If you do not feel pressure from the tennis ball, use a bigger ball, like a softball. This TBT is particularly easy to do in bed; just keep the ball and a book on your nightstand.

Precautions

Reposition the ball slightly if you feel a throbbing sensation or pulse coming from your leg when doing this exercise. That is simply your femoral artery doing its job.

TBT #7

Tennis Ball On Side Of Hip

This TBT will help release tension from the muscles and fascia that lie on the side of the hip.

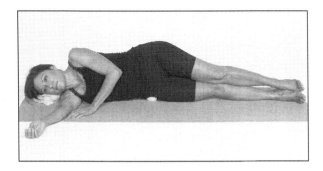

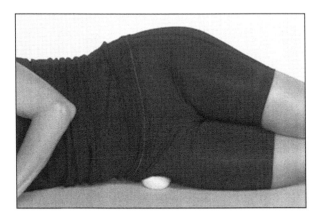

Where do I put the ball?

There are several muscles located on the side of the hip, such as the gluteus medius, gluteus minimus, and tensor fascia latae. Keeping these muscles free of tension and restrictions will help your legs, knees, hips, and lower back function and feel better.

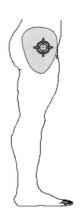

Do this TBT if you:

Stand a lot (especially with your weight propped on one hip); sit a lot; walk; run; do sports such as golf, tennis, snowboarding, ice-skating, snow-skiing, water-skiing, kayaking, or bowling; have back, hip, groin, or knee pain; had a knee replacement or surgery of the knee, back, hips, and/or ankle.

How do I do it?

Lie on your right side and place a tennis ball on the side of your hip (just above the top of your leg and just below your hip bone). When you find a sore spot, maintain pressure on it until it releases (5-10 seconds). Then move to the next spot. Repeat on the other hip. Do each side for about 1 to 2 minutes.

Tips

If the pressure is too great, simply angle your body so less of your weight is on top of the ball, or place a towel over the tennis ball for added cushioning. To make this TBT harder, angle your body so your hips are stacked directly over the ball.

Precautions

You may feel quite a bit of discomfort at first as the nerves in this area of the body are very sensitive. As such, do not use a hardball like a baseball, cricket ball, or lacrosse ball on this area; it will likely be too painful and may hurt the nerves.

TBT #8

Tennis Ball Under Back Of Leg

This TBT helps make the muscles and fascia on the back of the upper leg healthier and more flexible.

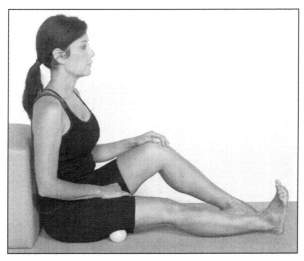

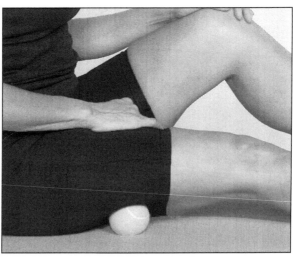

Where do I put the ball?

Your hamstring muscles are located on the back of your leg. They run the length of the upper leg from the middle of the butt to just below the knee. When they are limber and working correctly, they can help alleviate back, hip, knee, and neck pain.

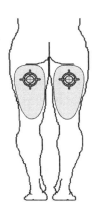

Do this TBT if you:

Stand a lot; sit a lot; garden; walk; run; bend over a lot; play sports like golf or tennis; have back, hip, knee, or neck pain; have ever torn your hamstrings; had a knee replacement; or surgery on the knee, back, hips, and/or ankle.

How do I do it?

Sit on the floor with your back against a wall. Place a tennis ball underneath the back of the upper thigh on one of your outstretched legs. Find a sore spot and maintain pressure on it until it releases (5-10 seconds). Then move to the next spot. Do each leg for about 1 to 2 minutes.

Tips

You can easily do this TBT while you watch TV—if you are sitting on a hard chair—or while lying in bed, by placing the ball on top of a book (to prevent it from sinking into the mattress). To make this exercise harder, flex your foot toward your shin and/or place the other leg on top of the one you are massaging to increase the pressure, or push the ball up into the leg by placing it on top of a book.

Precautions

When using a harder ball for this exercise, do not place direct pressure behind the knee.

TBT #9

Tennis Ball On Butt

This TBT helps recondition and bring blood supply to the muscles and fascia on the back of the hips, namely the glutes.

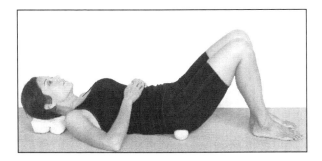

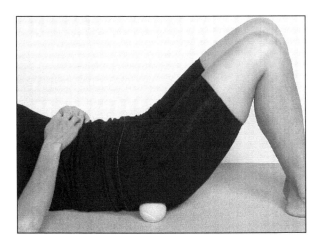

Where do I put the ball?

Your backside contains an amazing set of muscles called the gluteus maximus muscles. These big muscles and their surrounding fascia stabilize the end of the leg and hip socket and enable you to stand upright. Massaging this area keeps these tissues healthy and well-conditioned, which will contribute greatly to reducing lower back, hip, knee, and foot/ankle pain.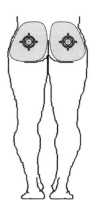

Do this TBT if you:

Sit a lot or for prolonged periods; prop your weight on one leg; garden, walk; run; bend over a lot; play any kind of sports; have back, hip, or knee pain; have had a knee or hip replacement; or surgery of the knee, back, hips, and/or ankle.

How do I do it?

Lie on the floor on your back with your knees bent. Place a tennis ball on the top part of your butt on one side of the body. Find a sore spot and maintain pressure on it until it releases (10-15 seconds). Then move to the next spot. When you have loosened all the muscles on one side of your butt, switch to the other side. Do each side for about 2 to 3 minutes.

Tips

You can do this exercise while you watch TV with your head supported by a pillow. It's also a great one to do while lying in bed—just remember to place the ball on a book first so it doesn't sink into the mattress. To make this TBT harder, place the ankle of the side you are massaging on top of the other knee to increase the pressure you feel from the ball.

Precautions

Do not place the ball on your tailbone or anywhere on the spine itself.

TBT #10

Tennis Ball On Lower Back

This TBT will help make the muscles and fascia of the lower back more flexible.

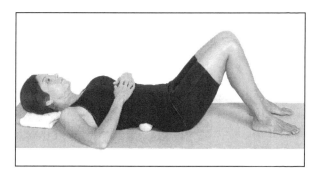

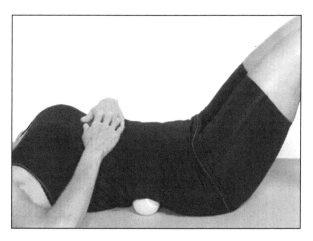

Where do I put the ball?

There are many muscles in the lower back on either side of your spine, between the top of the hips and the bottom of the rib cage (e.g., the lumbar erector spinae and the quadratus lumborum). Keeping these 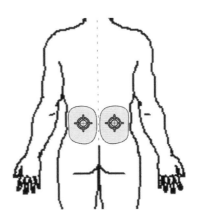 muscles healthy and flexible will enable your hips and lower back to move more freely and easily, which will decrease pain in these areas.

Do this TBT if you:

Sit a lot or for prolonged periods at a computer using a mouse; stand in high heels; walk; run; play any kind of sports; reach up over your head a lot; have back, hip, or knee pain; have had a hip replacement or surgery on the back or hips.

How do I do it?

Lie on the floor on your back with your knees bent. Place a tennis ball under one side of your spine in the space just above the back of your hips and below the bottom of your rib cage. Find a sore spot and maintain pressure on it until it releases (5-10 seconds). Then move to the next spot. When you have loosened all the muscles on one side of your lower back, switch to the other side. Do each side for about 1 to 2 minutes.

Tips

If the pressure is too great beside the spine, move the ball a few inches toward the outside of the body. To make this TBT harder, place the ankle of the side you are massaging on top of the other knee.

Precautions

Your two bottom ribs do not attach to the sternum, which makes them less stable than the other ribs, so be careful with the ball around this area. Also, do not place the ball directly on, or too close to the spine.

TBT #11

Tennis Ball(s) On Upper Back

This TBT will target the muscles that lie on either side of the spine in the upper back.

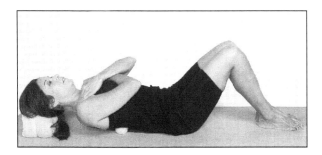

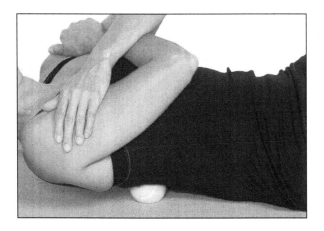

Where do I put the ball?

The muscles be-
side the spine in
your upper back
are called the
thoracic erector
spinae. They help
pull your torso
upright when
you are sitting or

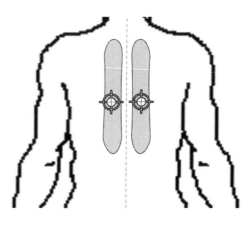

standing. Massaging these muscles will help release tension and keep them mobile, which will decrease pain in
the upper and lower back, and in the shoulders and neck.

Do this TBT if you:

Sit at a computer; play video games; drive a vehicle; stand
leaning over a table, counter, or sink; play sports where
you must bend over; engage in hobbies that require
close-up work, such as model building or needlepoint;
have back, shoulder, hip, knee, or foot pain; feel stressed
a lot; have breathing problems; have had abdominal surgery, upper or lower back surgery, or shoulder surgery.

How do I do it?

This TBT requires two tennis balls. Lie on the floor on your back with your knees bent and a large pillow under your head. Place a tennis ball on either side of your spine in line with the bottom of your shoulder blades. Bring your arms across your chest and hug yourself. Find a sore spot and maintain pressure on it until it releases (10-15 seconds). Then move the balls along your upper back to the next spot. When you need to move the balls up, simply scoot your butt and body down so that the balls roll up either side of your spine. Make sure to bring the pillow for your head with you each time you move. Do about 2 to 3 minutes on the entire area.

Tips

If you find it difficult to keep the balls in place, put them in a sock and tie a knot on the end to help keep them together. To make this TBT harder, flatten your lower back to the floor to increase pressure from the balls to the upper back, or use a smaller pillow for your head. To make it easier, use one ball at a time on either side of your spine.

Precautions

If you feel like your breathing is restricted when doing this exercise, then the pressure is too much for your body to be able to relax. Use a larger pillow to decrease the pressure you feel from the balls. As your body relaxes, you can gradually decrease the pillow height. Also, do not place the balls directly on your spine, but just on either side of it.

TBT #12

Tennis Ball On Back Of Shoulder

This TBT helps recondition the muscles on the upper back and the back of the shoulder.

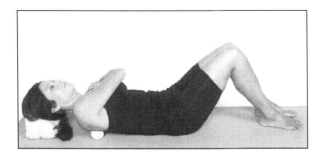

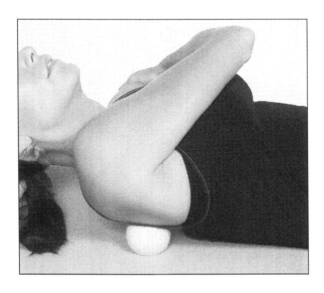

Where do I put the ball?

There are two large muscles in your upper back (the rhomboids and the trapezius) that run from the spine across to the shoulder blades. They help con-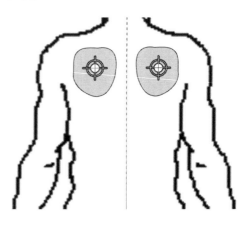trol movement of the spine and shoulder. Targeting these muscles to release tension and restrictions will help the upper and lower back, shoulders, neck, and arms feel better.

Do this TBT if you:

Sit at a computer; use your hands a lot for your work or hobbies; drive for long distances or periods; do a lot of cooking; carry heavy objects with your hands; play any kind of sports where you have to hold a piece of equipment in your hands; have back, shoulder, neck, hand, or wrist pain; feel stressed out a lot; have had upper or lower back surgery, shoulder surgery, and/or hand or wrist surgery.

How do I do it?

Lie on the floor on your back with your knees bent. Bring your right arm across your chest to hug your left shoulder/arm. Place a tennis ball under the right side of your upper back between the spine and your right shoulder blade. Find a sore spot and maintain pressure on it until it releases (10-15 seconds). Then move the ball to the next spot by scooting your butt and body slightly. When you have released all the sore spots on the right side, move the ball to the left side and repeat the process. Do each side for about 2 to 3 minutes.

Tips

To make this easier, put a towel over the ball to make it softer. This exercise can also be done standing up. Simply put a ball in a sock, hold on to the open end of the sock, and throw the ball over your shoulder. Then lean back against the wall to apply pressure to the desired area.

Precautions

When you do this exercise, you don't want your neck to arch backward so use a pillow to support your head.

TBT #13

Tennis Ball On Front Of Shoulder

This TBT helps recondition the muscles and fascia on the front of the shoulder and chest.

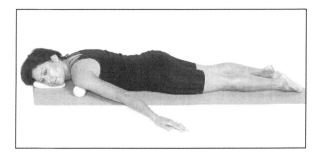

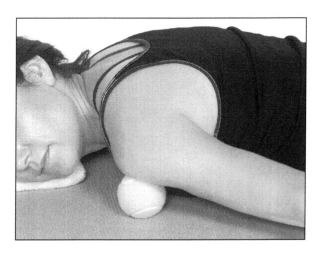

Where do I put the ball?

There are several muscles on the front of the shoulder (the pectorals, the deltoid, and the origin of the biceps of the arm) that affect the function of the ribcage,

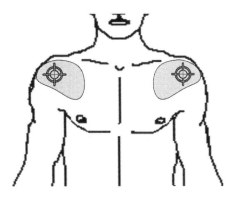

upper back, shoulders and arms. Releasing tension and restrictions from these muscles can make your shoulders and arms function better, reduce pain in your upper back and neck, and enable you to breathe easier.

Do this TBT if you:

Sit at a computer; sleep on your side or stomach; use your hands to work or for hobbies; drive a lot or for long periods; cook a lot; play any sport where you have to hold a piece of equipment in your hands; play a musical instrument; have back, shoulder, neck, hand, or wrist pain; feel stressed a lot; have had upper or lower back surgery, shoulder surgery, and/or hand or wrist surgery.

How do I do it?

Lie face down on the floor and extend your left arm straight out from your body just below shoulder height, with your palm down. Use the other hand to place a tennis ball underneath the front of your left shoulder and upper chest. Find a sore spot and maintain pressure on it until it releases (5-10 seconds). Then move to the next spot. Repeat on the right side. Do each side for about 1 to 2 minutes.

Tips

If you feel discomfort in your neck with your head turned to one side, turn your head the other way.

Precautions

Use a small pillow to support your head to keep your neck in line with your spine.

TBT #14

Tennis Ball On Abdominals

This TBT helps recondition and rejuvenate the muscles and fascia that lie on the front of the torso below your sternum.

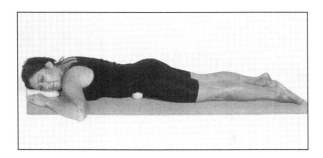

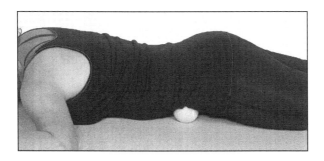

Where do I put the ball?

The abdominal muscles (rectus abdominis, transverse abdominis, and obliques) and the hip flexor muscles (psoas minor, psoas major, and iliacus) are just some of the important tissues you are going to make healthier with this TBT.

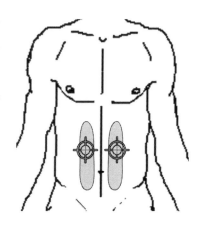

Keeping the muscles and fascia in your abdominal area bendable and twistable will decrease hip, upper and lower back, knee, butt, and groin pain.

Do this TBT if you:

Run, walk, squat or lunge; do sit-ups or crunches; play sports; have back or knee pain; had back surgery; feel stressed a lot; have breathing problems; had abdominal, knee, hip, or ankle surgery.

How do I do it?

Lie on the floor face down. Place a tennis ball between your stomach and the floor just below the bottom of your rib cage (i.e., sternum), to the right of your bellybutton (but not on your ribs). Find a sore spot and maintain pressure on it until it releases (5-10 seconds). Then move to the next spot by scooting your body up so the ball moves down. Do this all along your abdomen, past your bellybutton to the top of your hips. Then repeat the process on left side. Do each side for about 1 to 2 minutes.

Tips

Turn the leg on the side you are massaging inward so the top of your foot rests on the ground. This will help stretch the deeper hip flexor muscles. To make this harder, use a new tennis ball to increase pressure on the area. To make it easier, place a towel over the ball.

Precautions

If you have had abdominal surgery in the past, be gentle as you roll the ball over the scar. Also, if you feel a pulse under the ball when doing this exercise, move the ball slightly off that spot. That is normal; it's simply your femoral artery pulsing.

TBT #15

Tennis Ball On Forearm

This TBT helps release tension from the muscles and fascia of the upper and lower arm and the wrist/hand.

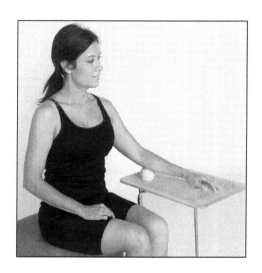

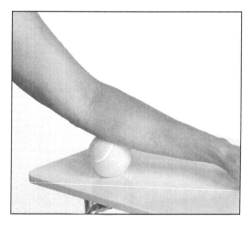

Where do I put the ball?

There are many muscles in your forearm that control the wrist and fingers. These muscles and their surrounding fascia affect the function of the hand, wrist, arm, shoulder, and even the back. Releasing tension and restrictions in the tissues of the lower arm can reduce pain in all these areas.

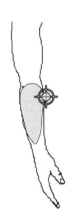

Do this TBT if you:

Type or use handheld electronic devices; do hand-focused hobbies such as painting or knitting; do a lot of handwriting; do exercises that require you to grip weights or other pieces of equipment; carry or lift heavy objects; garden, drive, or cook a lot; play sports where you have to hold a piece of equipment in your hands; play a musical instrument; have hand, wrist, back, shoulder, or neck pain; feel stressed a lot; have had or currently have carpal tunnel syndrome; or have had any surgery on the shoulder and/or hand or wrist.

How do I do it?

Sit on a chair with your arm extended—palm down—over a desk, countertop, or table. Place a tennis ball underneath your forearm and find a sore spot. Maintain pressure on it until it releases (5-10 seconds). Then move to the next spot. Do both the underside and top of your forearm (by turning your hand palm up). Do each arm for about 1 to 2 minutes.

Tips

If you are right-handed, do the right side more. If you're left-handed, do the left side more. You can also do this exercise lying on the ground with your arm outstretched to the side.

Precautions

Do not place a hard ball on the tendons near the underside of the wrist.

TBT #16

Tennis Ball On Back Of Neck

This TBT will help release tension from the muscles and fascia on the back of the neck and top of shoulders.

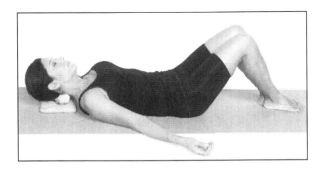

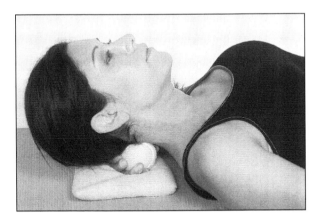

Where do I put the ball?

There are muscles on ei-
ther side of the back of
your neck called the cer-
vical erector spinae. They
help keep your head on
straight. Target these muscles to release excess tension from the head, neck,
and shoulders.

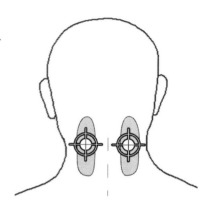

Do this TBT if you:

Sit at a computer; watch television or play video games;
read, drive, or do a lot of cooking; have neck, jaw, back,
or shoulder pain; feel stressed out a lot; grind or grit your
teeth; have frequent tension headaches; or have had neck
or shoulder surgery.

How do I do it?

Lie on the floor on your back with your knees bent. Cup
a tennis ball in your left hand. Place the ball behind your
head to the right side of your neck. Find a sore spot and
maintain pressure on it until it releases (5-10 seconds).
Then move to the next spot. Do this on both sides of the
back of your neck. Do each side for about 1 to 2 minutes.

Tips

If you have trouble reaching behind your head, place the tennis ball on a towel on top of a book and then rest your neck on the ball. To make this harder, gently tuck your chin to your chest and push the back of your head down into the floor/ball. To make it easier, use a pillow to support your head.

Precautions

Do not bring the ball around to the front or side of your neck where your carotid artery and other fragile structures are located.

TBT Common Ailments Guide

If you're still not sure which TBTs are right for you, simply refer to the guide below to see which ones are recommended for various common ailments. The amount of TBTs you will choose for your specific condition or situation will vary, but all possible techniques for each issue have been listed to help get you started.

Foot, Ankle, and Heel Pain

(such as plantar fasciitis, Achilles tendonitis, Morten's neuroma, heel spurs, arthritis, neuropathy, bunions, and hammer toes)

TBT #1	Tennis Ball Under Foot
TBT #2	Tennis Ball Under Calf
TBT #3	Tennis Ball Side Of Calf
TBT #5	Tennis Ball On Side Of Leg
TBT #9	Tennis Ball On Butt
TBT #10	Tennis Ball On Lower Back
TBT #11	Tennis Ball(s) On Upper Back

Leg and Knee Pain

(such as calf pain, patella femoral syndrome, chondro-malacia patella, shin splints, meniscus injuries, ligament strains and muscle sprains, bursitis, tendonitis, neuropathy, arthritis, and ITB syndrome)

TBT #1	Tennis Ball Under Foot
TBT #2	Tennis Ball Under Calf
TBT #3	Tennis Ball Side Of Calf
TBT #4	Tennis Ball On Front Of Thigh
TBT #5	Tennis Ball On Side Of Leg
TBT #6	Tennis Ball On Inner Thigh
TBT #7	Tennis Ball On Side Of Hip
TBT #8	Tennis Ball Under Back Of Leg
TBT #9	Tennis Ball On Butt
TBT #11	Tennis Ball(s) On Upper Back

Lower Back, Hip, and Abdominal Pain

(such as sciatica, piriformis syndrome, bursitis, disc issues, muscle spasms, sacroiliac joint dysfunction, ligament strains and muscle sprains, arthritis, and irritable bowel syndrome)

TBT #1	Tennis Ball Under Foot
TBT #2	Tennis Ball Under Calf
TBT #4	Tennis Ball On Front Of Thigh
TBT #5	Tennis Ball On Side Of Leg
TBT #7	Tennis Ball On Side Of Hip

TBT #9   Tennis Ball On Butt
TBT #10 Tennis Ball On Lower Back
TBT #11 Tennis Ball(s) On Upper Back
TBT #12 Tennis Ball On Back Of Shoulder
TBT #13 Tennis Ball On Front Of Shoulder
TBT #14 Tennis Ball On Abdominals
TBT #16 Tennis Ball On Back Of Neck

Upper Back Pain, Arm/Wrist, and Shoulder Pain

(such as rotator cuff problems, frozen shoulder, carpal tunnel syndrome, tennis and golfer's elbow, arthritis, tendonitis, ligament strains and muscle sprains, neuropathy, and thoracic outlet syndrome)

TBT #1   Tennis Ball Under Foot
TBT #9   Tennis Ball On Butt
TBT #11 Tennis Ball(s) On Upper Back
TBT #12 Tennis Ball On Back Of Shoulder
TBT #13 Tennis Ball On Front Of Shoulder
TBT #14 Tennis Ball On Abdominals
TBT #15 Tennis Ball On Forearm
TBT #16 Tennis Ball On Back Of Neck

Neck, Head, and Jaw Pain

(such as muscle spasms, tension headaches, ligament strains and muscle sprains, TMJ, arthritis, neuropathy and disc issues)

TBT #1	Tennis Ball Under Foot
TBT #9	Tennis Ball On Butt
TBT #11	Tennis Ball(s) On Upper Back
TBT #12	Tennis Ball On Back Of Shoulder
TBT #13	Tennis Ball On Front Of Shoulder
TBT #14	Tennis Ball On Abdominals
TBT #15	Tennis Ball On Forearm
TBT #16	Tennis Ball On Back Of Neck

Other chronic issues such as:

Fibromyalgia

TBT #1	Tennis Ball Under Foot
TBT #2	Tennis Ball Under Calf
TBT #4	Tennis Ball On Front Of Thigh
TBT #5	Tennis Ball On Side Of Leg
TBT #9	Tennis Ball On Butt
TBT #10	Tennis Ball On Lower Back
TBT #11	Tennis Ball(s) On Upper Back
TBT #12	Tennis Ball On Back Of Shoulder

TBT #13 Tennis Ball On Front Of Shoulder

TBT #14 Tennis Ball On Abdominals

TBT #16 Tennis Ball On Back Of Neck

Asthma

TBT #9 Tennis Ball On Butt

TBT #10 Tennis Ball On Lower Back

TBT #11 Tennis Ball(s) On Upper Back

TBT #12 Tennis Ball On Back Of Shoulder

TBT #13 Tennis Ball On Front Of Shoulder

TBT #14 Tennis Ball On Abdominals

TBT #16 Tennis Ball On Back Of Neck

Chronic Stress and Fatigue

TBT #1 Tennis Ball Under Foot

TBT #2 Tennis Ball Under Calf

TBT #9 Tennis Ball On Butt

TBT #10 Tennis Ball On Lower Back

TBT #11 Tennis Ball(s) On Upper Back

TBT #12 Tennis Ball On Back Of Shoulder

TBT #13 Tennis Ball On Front Of Shoulder

TBT #14 Tennis Ball On Abdominals

TBT #16 Tennis Ball On Back Of Neck

Chapter 5

Other Tips To Soothe Your Back Pain

Doing The BioMechanics Method's Tennis Ball Techniques is one of the most inexpensive, efficient, and effective ways to ease your back pain. However, making just a few adjustments to your everyday habits can also go a long way toward relieving your aches and pains, while promoting a healthier back. In this chapter, I would like to share some extra tips that have helped my clients see even greater results in getting rid of persistent pain. But before I do, I have to emphasize one thing about this entire program, and it's absolutely critical

115

to your overall success.

Progress gradually. Don't overdo it!

Think about if you were going to run a marathon. You wouldn't just show up on the morning of the race and try to run 26.2 miles without training, would you? Of course not. You would start slowly by walking or jogging short distances, and then build up over time to longer distances. By the time race day arrived, you would be prepared to make it to the finish line without injuring yourself.

That's how you should approach the techniques and tips in this program. Don't start doing *all* the TBTs for an hour a day, and following *all* the tips in this chapter from the get-go. Pick a few TBTs that are best for your needs and introduce them gradually to your daily routine, spending just 5-10 minutes *total* per day. Slowly adjust a few of your everyday habits. If you try to do too much too fast, you may end up overdoing it and slow your overall progress.

Take my dad, for example. I remember when I was a kid he developed plantar fasciitis, which causes pain in the bottom of the foot. It got to the point where he could barely walk anymore. He went to see a foot doctor, who gave him a prescription for arch supports and told him they would take care of the problem. Without question, my dad eagerly placed them in his shoes and proceeded through the day as normal. He went to work, played golf, and then took our dog on a long walk.

The following day he was in agony, complaining about "that crazy foot doctor who doesn't know what he's talking about!" But it wasn't the doctor's fault, and it wasn't the arch supports' fault either. It was my dad who had simply overdone it. The arch supports provided a new sensation for his body. His muscles, fascia, ligaments, tendons, and bones had to adapt to the new shoe inserts and needed time to do so.

Keep in mind that the TBTs and tips here are new to your body and may be waking up muscles that have been asleep for a long time. Give your body time to adjust. This will help ensure that you get the greatest relief for your pain, and increases the likelihood you will continue with the program, which is key for long-term relief. With this in mind, take note of the following simple changes you can make to your everyday habits and routines.

Aim For Better Posture

Pay attention to your posture throughout the day; you will start to notice little habits that have become automatic. These habits may be adding to your aching back. By making just a few slight alterations, you can start improving your overall musculoskeletal health, which will reduce your pain.

Sitting at Your Computer

When it comes to sitting at your computer, think variety. Contrary to what ergonomics experts claim, there is no ideal way to sit because sitting at a computer for prolonged periods is simply not ideal for your body. There is no perfect chair height, no magic angle for your hands and wrists that will stave off aches and pains. Instead of searching for the *one* best seating position, vary your seating position and do it often. When your body is stuck in one single position—even if it's the most ergonomically correct one—for hours, you end up using the same muscles in the same way all the time and neglecting other muscles, all of which adds up to pain and dysfunction.

To minimize computer-related issues:

- Alter your seat height throughout the day.
- Switch to using the mouse with your non-dominant hand from time to time.
- Change the height of your computer monitor (put a book under it sometimes).
- Try different seats—office chair, stool, stability ball.

- Change your keyboard height.
- Make the text size on your computer bigger so you don't have to lean forward to read it.
- Use voice recognition software so you can stand while working at your computer rather than sitting and typing.
- Take lots of mini-breaks—stand up and walk around often.
- If you're using a laptop or tablet and you want to put it on your lap, place a pillow on your legs under the device to avoid having to round your back to see it.

Sitting in Your Car

Want to know a great trick that will force you to sit upright while driving? All you have to do is sit up tall and adjust your rear-view mirror for ideal viewing. Whenever you notice you can't see properly out the back window, *don't* change the mirror. It's likely that if you can no longer see well with the way the mirror is angled, you've started to slouch. So instead of fixing the mirror, fix your posture.

Sitting on the Couch

Remember when I talked about variety? Keep it in mind when you're on the couch too. Most of us always sit on the same side of the couch and lean on the armrest, which creates problems. Try sitting on the opposite side, or lying down from time to time, or sit in an armchair. You can even sit on a stability ball sometimes while watching TV, or try standing up every time a commercial comes on. If you like to eat your meals while on the couch, put a pillow on your lap under the plate so you don't have to round your back quite so much to eat.

Walking

Walking seems so simple; you just put one foot in front of the other, right? So why do so many of us get it wrong? In prehistoric times, we walked barefoot over rugged terrain, which required the muscles in our feet to work hard to stabilize our bodies and prevent falls. In our modern-day society, we protect our feet with shoes and have created flat and smooth surfaces for walking. The problem with this is the muscles in your feet no longer need to do much work to keep you stable. As you now know, this means those muscles go to sleep, which leads to a chain of dysfunction that travels up to your calves, knees, and hips.

The solution is to wake up those muscles in your feet by reintroducing them to uneven surfaces. I'm not suggesting you suddenly go barefoot everywhere, but you may want to try walking on different surfaces when you can, such as cobblestones, grass, or dirt trails. Just don't go from spending your days on concrete or carpeted floors to doing a 12-mile hike with no shoes. Wake up your foot muscles gradually!

Standing

When you're on your feet, it's important to notice how you tend to stand. Do you usually shift your weight from side to side? Do you typically jut one hip out? Do you often lean on a counter, against a wall, or with your hand on a desk? All of these are signs that your body isn't comfortable standing up with good posture, and that can contribute to an aching back.

To improve the health of your back, gradually increase the amount of time you spend standing without shifting your weight, sticking one hip out, or leaning on things. And remember, these habits have taken a lifetime to develop, so don't expect to change them instantaneously.

Sleeping

Have you ever woken up in the morning with a sore back or neck and assumed you must have slept in a funny position? You could be right. Considering that we spend six, seven, eight, or more hours snoozing, the way we sleep can play a major role in causing aches and pains.

- **If you're a back sleeper:** If you sleep on your back with your legs straight, your lower back will likely overarch. After a period of many hours, this can lead to soreness. To avoid overarching, place a large pillow under your knees. This bent-knee position will help decrease the arch in your lower back as you sleep. Also, use a small pillow under your head so it does not angle forward of your spine.

- **If you're a side sleeper:** When you sleep on your side, you place your body weight on top of one shoulder and arm and probably round the other shoulder forward too, to bring your top hand onto the bed. You also typically let your top leg rest on the bottom one or on the bed, which pulls on your pelvis, which then pulls on your back. To minimize problems caused by side sleeping, extend your bottom arm out straight away from your body, rest your top arm on your top hip, and use a body pillow or a towel between your legs to help keep them hip-width apart. Also choose a pillow for your head that aligns your neck with your spine.

- **If you sleep on your stomach:** Sleeping on

your stomach is the worst position if you have back pain. It causes you to overarch your lower back, round your shoulders, and twist your neck to one side. This means that if you also spend your day hunched over your computer, you have bad posture for almost 24 hours a day. If at all possible, try to avoid sleeping face down.

Find the Best Footwear for Your Needs

Did you know that wearing certain types of shoes can lead to back pain? High-heels are a major culprit. They raise your heels off the ground, which tilts your pelvis forward and causes your lower back to overarch. That makes your muscles—especially those in your back—work extra hard to keep you upright while you are standing or walking. If you wear running shoes when you are not running, they may be hurting your back as well. Many types of athletic shoes are higher in the heel than in the toe, which makes them high-heeled, which causes problems.

Don't think that sandals or flip-flops are any better since they don't have a heel. Your feet slide around in them, which forces all the muscles, fascia, tendons, and ligaments above your feet to concentrate more on keeping the shoes on when you are walking than on propelling you forward.

Other shoe issues include footwear that is too tight in the toebox. If your toes are all scrunched up, it decreases the surface area of your foot. That makes your muscles work harder to keep you balanced. The back end of your shoe can cause problems too, especially if your heel tends to slip in and out of the back of your shoes. This makes everything above your foot work overtime.

Do your back a favor by following these footwear tips:

- Try to wear neutral-soled shoes (shoes that aren't higher in the heel than the toes).
- Choose shoes that have enough space at the front for your toes to spread out.
- Choose shoes that do not slip on the heel.

What About Orthotics or Arch Supports?

If you're like my dad, you may try orthotics at some point. They are inserts that go inside your shoes to provide support for your foot. If so, just be sure to introduce them gradually rather than overdoing it. As your muscles and fascia get healthier and your body gets into better alignment, use the arch supports less and less. You may eventually find that you don't need to use them at all anymore.

Accessorize Without Hurting Your Back

All of those seemingly handy devices you tote around on

a daily basis can really do a number on your back. Here are just a few examples. Talking on your cell phone can cause you to tilt your head to one side, which tips you off balance and makes your back work harder. Texting makes you round your shoulders and spine forward. Wearing a purse on the same side all the time bends your back to one side. Putting a fat wallet in your back pocket and then sitting on it causes an imbalance in your hips and spine. Holding a dog leash tautly in one hand can prevent you from swinging your arms as you walk, which puts more pressure on your lower back. The list goes on.

To help ease your pain, follow these practical hints:

- Use hands-free communication devices whenever possible.
- Trade your purse for a backpack that you can wear over both shoulders.
- When walking the dog, change the leash from side to side or consider one that ties around your waist.
- Don't carry your wallet in your back pocket.
- Don't put heavy items in your front pockets.

Reduce Your Stress to Reduce Your Back Pain

In prehistoric times, humans experienced stress when they came upon a physical threat, such as a vicious wild animal. When faced with this kind of stress, the body goes into a fight-or-flight response because it believes it needs to protect itself against a threat. This causes the muscles to tighten in preparation for action—either running away from the animal or fighting off an attack. After the threat is gone, the body's muscles relax and go back to normal.

In today's world, stress comes from all kinds of perceived "threats": your mother-in-law coming to visit, disturbing events on the nightly news, or feeling like you can't get out from under the barrage of emails in your inbox. This stress creates the same physical response in the body, causing muscles to tense up. The problem for many of us is that this everyday stress never lets up, so our muscles never get to relax. This muscle tension can put pressure on nerves and cause pain.

Thoughts and perceptions that cause psychological stress are one of the leading causes of back pain. But don't just take my word for it. A number of independent studies in Sweden, the United States, and Finland have shown direct connections between mental stress and the experience of physical pain. The bottom line? Thinking stressful thoughts results in physical responses in the body that can lead to back pain.

If you become conscious of the things that cause you stress, you can attempt to reduce those things or control your response to them. You can also use stress reduction techniques—deep breathing, meditation, and more—to help minimize stress and the muscle tension that accompanies it. This can help alleviate the pressure on sensitive nerves so you can ease your pain.

Reduce Your Level of Stress About Whether the TBTs Will Work For You

Have you already tried everything to alleviate your back pain without relief? Are you worried that the exercises in this book aren't going to work either? These types of thoughts may actually reduce the likelihood that the TBTs will work for you. They may cause you to over-react and either give up too soon or do an unrealistic number or amount of the techniques each day.

If you give up, I can guarantee you aren't going to reduce your aches and pains. And if you do too much, you may not be able to keep up the pace for very long. As such, you may quit doing the exercises altogether. Then you will just go back to your back pain again.

The key to lasting success and pain relief is to introduce the TBTs gradually and set realistic goals. Aim to make the exercises a lifetime habit, so start with just 5-10 minutes a day. After a while, if you want to do more, build up to 10-15 minutes a day. All in all, I wouldn't recommend doing more than 30 minutes a day of the TBTs, even after you have mastered all the moves. The other key to keeping back pain at bay for the long-term is having realistic expectations. As I mentioned earlier, your back pain didn't happen overnight, and you won't get rid of the underlying causes overnight. Be patient and enjoy the daily improvements in how you feel along the way.

Reduce Your Level of Stress About Your Back Pain

Does your back pain cause you additional stress? Do you stress about the activities you will no longer be able to do if your back pain continues to get worse? Do you imagine a day when you can barely get out of bed or you'll have to walk hunched over because you can't straighten up? Do you search online to see what you're headed for if your sore back doesn't improve? These kinds of thoughts are not helping you get better, so stop stressing about your back!

If you can't control your compulsion to search on the Internet, try to avoid websites that offer nothing but worst-case scenarios. Websites that recommend drug-based treatments or surgical solutions for your back pain are typically designed to increase your anxiety so you will panic and buy their products.

Most importantly, I urge you to stop doing those things you know are causing your back to hurt more. For example, if your back always aches when you do a certain exercise, say when you jog, try to limit the amount of time you spend jogging while you introduce the TBTs to help realign your body and improve the health of your muscles and fascia.

This was a hard lesson for my client Bill, who came to me for help with his back pain. He told me that his back hurt whenever he played basketball or did ab crunches, so I recommended he give up the basketball and crunches—just for a brief period while we addressed his back issues. A few weeks into the program, Bill wasn't getting any better, which is highly unusual if someone is doing the TBTs regularly. It turned out Bill was still playing basketball and doing those crunches. Eventually he admitted he was afraid that if he didn't do his regular activities—even for a few weeks—he would put on weight.

That's when we had a heart to heart about his priorities. Was he more interested in curing his back pain so he could enjoy the activities he loves (and keep weight off) for the rest of his life, or more concerned about possibly gaining a couple of pounds until he resumed his activities pain-free? Ultimately Bill decided that, in the long run, having a healthy back would be more helpful in keeping his weight down, so he skipped the activities he knew were harmful for his back and focused on his TBTs. To his surprise, he didn't gain a single pound, and he was back to playing basketball and doing his gym routine without pain sooner than he expected.

If you're like Bill, you may be fretting about giving up certain activities, even on a temporary basis. However, rest assured, doing the TBTs will improve the chances you will get to continue doing the things you love to do for years to come, rather than having to give them up permanently due to pain.

I have worked with a lot of clients who worry about all the things they might not be able to do in the future if their back pain persists. What if I can no longer work or travel? What if I can't play the piano anymore? What if I can't take my dog for a walk? If you find yourself fretting about the future, focus instead on what you can do *now* to help your problem, like the TBTs. Taking action to improve your back pain puts you in control of the problem rather than feeling victimized by it. That simple attitude adjustment can go a long way toward boosting your mood, improving your outlook, and ultimately easing your pain.

Conclusion

Your aching back is basically sending you an urgent message that your muscles, fascia, tendons, ligaments, and bones aren't working the way they're supposed to. They're either slacking off, out of alignment, or working overtime. It's up to you to respond to this message.

As you have seen in this book, your body works together as a whole, so in order to successfully eliminate your pain, you can't just focus on fixing your back. You have to address all the parts that aren't working well. And you have to consider all the things you do throughout the course of the day (and night) that might be contributing to your body's dysfunction. To get everything back up to speed and to find lasting relief, you need to:

- Choose to use the techniques in this book. Do the TBTs in addition to making small changes to your everyday habits and patterns.
- Be patient. Your body didn't get out of whack overnight, so don't expect overnight results.
- Be diligent. Make the TBTs a part of your daily routine, just like brushing your teeth.
- Maintain a positive outlook. If you approach something with the mental attitude that it is not going to work, then it won't! You have control of your mindset, so set yourself up to succeed.

Your pain may have you feeling discouraged, and after reading all the information in this book, you may be feeling overwhelmed. That's natural because it is a lot to take in. So start today with these simple steps:

1. Get a tennis ball.
2. Figure out where you feel pain the most, and what you are doing that makes the pain feel worse.
3. Choose TBTs to address the areas where you feel pain, and stop doing the things that make your pain worse until the TBTs start to take effect.

I would wish you luck with alleviating your back pain, but if you follow the strategies outlined in this book, you are not going to need it.

About the Author

Justin Price is a biomechanics specialist, expert in corrective exercise, and creator of The BioMechanics Method®. His assessment and exercise techniques are widely used by health and fitness professionals around the world to help people eliminate chronic pain. Justin's techniques have also been featured in *Time Magazine*, *Newsweek*, *The New York Times*, *The Wall Street Journal*, *The Los Angeles Times*, *The Chicago Tribune*, *Tennis Magazine*, *Men's Health*, *Arthritis Today*, and on WebMD and Discovery Health.

Date Due

BRODART, CO.   Cat. No. 23-233   Printed in U.S.A.

19241419R00083

Made in the USA
San Bernardino, CA
18 February 2015